YOUR PAINFUL SHOULDER

Dr Daniel Silver
Your Painful Shoulder

All rights reserved
Copyright © 2024 by Dr Daniel Silver

Published by Spines
ISBN 979-8-89569-301-8

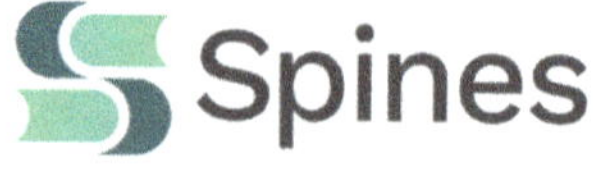

YOUR PAINFUL SHOULDER

A PATIENT GUIDE TO DIAGNOSIS AND TREATMENT

DANIEL M. SILVER, M.D.

ORTHOPEDIC SURGEON

CONTENTS

INTRODUCTION

In active society there are many sports injuries, activities, and other conditions that affect all of our bodies and especially our joints. As an orthopedic surgeon I have seen thousands of patients of all ages. Most people have no understanding of their injuries or the cause of the pain they are suffering.

My purpose in writing this book is from the perspective of an Orthopedic Surgeon practicing 43 years to inform athletes and others of the damage that has been done both anatomically and physiologically to their bodies.

Functions have been lost. My goal is to show you how we correct these things using the most conservative methods first and then progressing to surgery if necessary. It can't be emphasized enough that physical therapy is extremely important from the beginning of treatment to the end.

X-ray and MRI imaging that is necessary for diagnosis. After describing how an accurate diagnosis is achieved, I outline a plan for conservative treatment, therapy, and in many cases surgical correction of the injuries or conditions.

It is my hope that this book will inform the reader sufficiently to make informed decisions with their orthopedic surgeon and other providers. I will detail, in many cases, the surgical procedures as well as the follow up care and physical therapy necessary for optimal results. Now let's look at the anatomy involved.

This book is the first in a series of body areas to be covered by Dr. Silver and is focused on the shoulder joint. The anatomy of the bones, muscles, ligaments, plus neurovascular structures will be illustrated and discussed in detail. Then step- by- step we will take various diagnoses, explain them in detail and cover the choices of treatment including outcomes, risks, and potential complications.

In this book I will answer questions that you should ask of your orthopedic surgeon for example:

1. What is the exact nature of my shoulder problem?
2. Why is surgery being recommended?
3. What are the specific risks and benefits of the recommended surgery?
4. What is the expected recovery timeline?
5. What kind of rehabilitation will be necessary?
6. What are the potential complications and how common are they?
7. What are the alternatives to surgery and what are their success rates?

Welcome to!

Your Painful Shoulder

A Patient Guide to Diagnosis and Treatment

1 SHOULDER ANATOMY AND BIOMECHANICS

THE SHOULDER IS A COMPLEX JOINT WITH VARIOUS STRUCTURES working together to provide a wide range of motion. The shoulder helps place the arm and the hand in the proper position in space for gripping or lifting objects with the hand. Below is an explanation of the anatomy of the shoulder region followed by a discussion of the biomechanics and function of the shoulder.

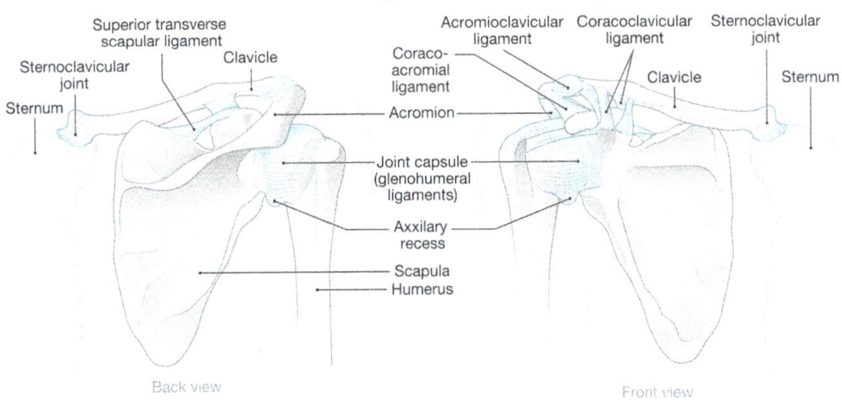

Fig. 1.1 Bony Anatomy

BONES

1. **Clavicle** (also called the collarbone):The bone that connects the shoulder blade to the sternum or breastbone. It forms a connection from the shoulder area to the center of the skeleton via the rib cage.
2. **Scapula** (also called the shoulder blade): The triangular bone that sits on the back of the rib cage and has many muscle attachments integral to the movement of the shoulder. It also has an articular (joint contacting) surface called the glenoid which serves as the socket portion of the ball and socket arrangement with the humeral head for rotation of the arm. There is also a bony projection at the point of the shoulder called the acromion that has many muscle attachments such as the Deltoid muscle.
3. **Humerus:** The bone of the upper arm. It has a ball at the top called the head of the humerus. There are many muscle attachments to this bone that rotate and abduct (lift away from body) the arm from the side. There is also a very smooth articular surface on the head of the humerus which moves as a part of the ball and socket joint with the glenoid (the cup on the scapula)

JOINTS

1. **Glenohumeral Joint**: The ball-and-socket joint where the humerus fits into the scapula. This is the main joint of the shoulder that allows 360` movement.
2. **Acromioclavicular (AC) Joint**: The joint where the clavicle meets the acromion (a part of the scapula).
3. **Sternoclavicular (SC) Joint**: The joint where the clavicle meets the sternum of the ribcage.
4. **Scapulothoracic Joint**: A functional joint where the scapula glides over the ribcage.

MUSCLES

1. **Deltoid**: The large, triangular muscle covering the shoulder joint.
2. **Rotator Cuff Muscles**: Four muscles (Supraspinatus, Infraspinatus, Teres Minor, and Subscapularis) that stabilize the shoulder.
3. **Trapezius**: A large muscle extending down the back and neck like a shawl draped over the shoulders and upper back.
4. **Pectoralis Major**: The chest muscle that helps with shoulder movements in the forward direction.

TENDONS AND LIGAMENTS

Shoulder anatomy. Rotator cuff muscles

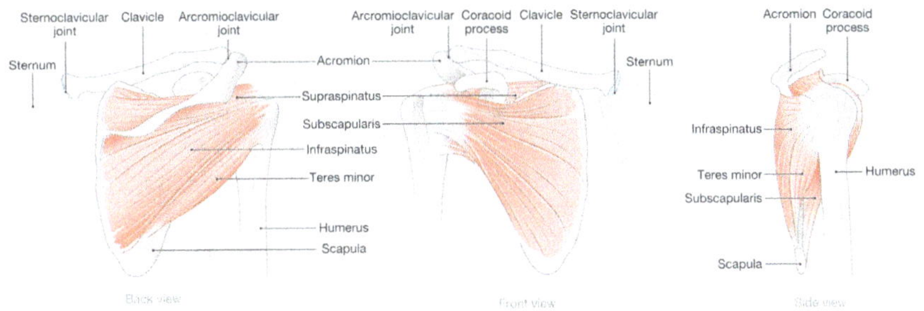

Sternoclavicular joint · Clavicle · Acromioclavicular joint · Sternum · Acromion · Supraspinatus · Subscapularis · Infraspinatus · Teres minor · Humerus · Scapula · Back view

Acromioclavicular joint · Coracoid process · Clavicle · Sternoclavicular joint · Sternum · Front view

Acromion · Coracoid process · Infraspinatus · Teres minor · Subscapularis · Humerus · Scapula · Side view

Fig.1. 2 Muscles, Tendons, and Ligaments

1. **Coracoclavicular Ligament**: Connects the coracoid process of the scapula to the clavicle. This ligament is attached to the coracoid process of the scapula and connects to the underside of the clavicle in two parts: the coronoid and the trapezoid. These two portions contribute at least 50 to 60% of the strength of the acromioclavicular stability.
2. **Acromioclavicular Ligament**: Connects the distal end of the clavicle to the acromion which is a portion of the

scapula. This ligament contributes 40 to 50% of the strength of the acromioclavicular stability. In an injury such as a fall or impact on the shoulder joint, this ligament tears first in an AC separation before the coracoclavicular ligament tears.

3. **Glenohumeral Ligaments:** Stabilize the glenohumeral joint. These are thickenings in the capsule of the shoulder joint. The main thickenings of the capsule are the superior, middle, and inferior glenohumeral ligaments.

4. **Coracoacromial Ligament:** Connects the coracoid process to the acromion and provides anterior stability to the humeral head in the glenoid fossa.

5. **Rotator Cuff Tendons:** Include the tendons of four muscles (supraspinatus, infraspinatus, teres minor, and subscapularis) that stabilize the shoulder joint and allow for rotation and lifting movements.

6. **Biceps Tendon:** The tendon of the long head of the biceps brachii also contributes to shoulder stability as it passes through the bicipital groove of the humerus.

BURSAE

Shoulder anatomy. Bursae and muscles

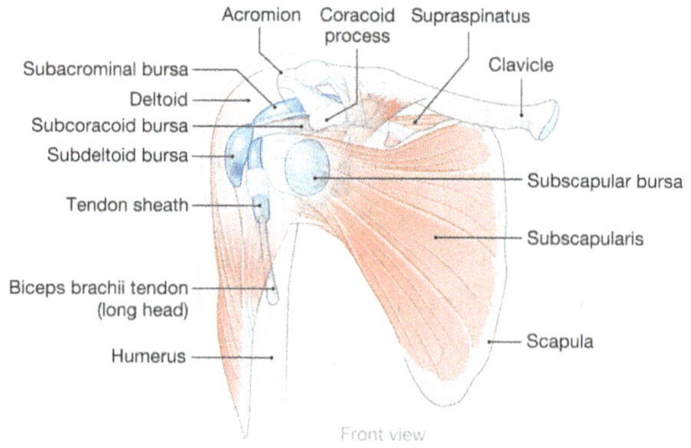

Fig. 1.3.1 Subacromial Bursa

SHOULDER JOINT

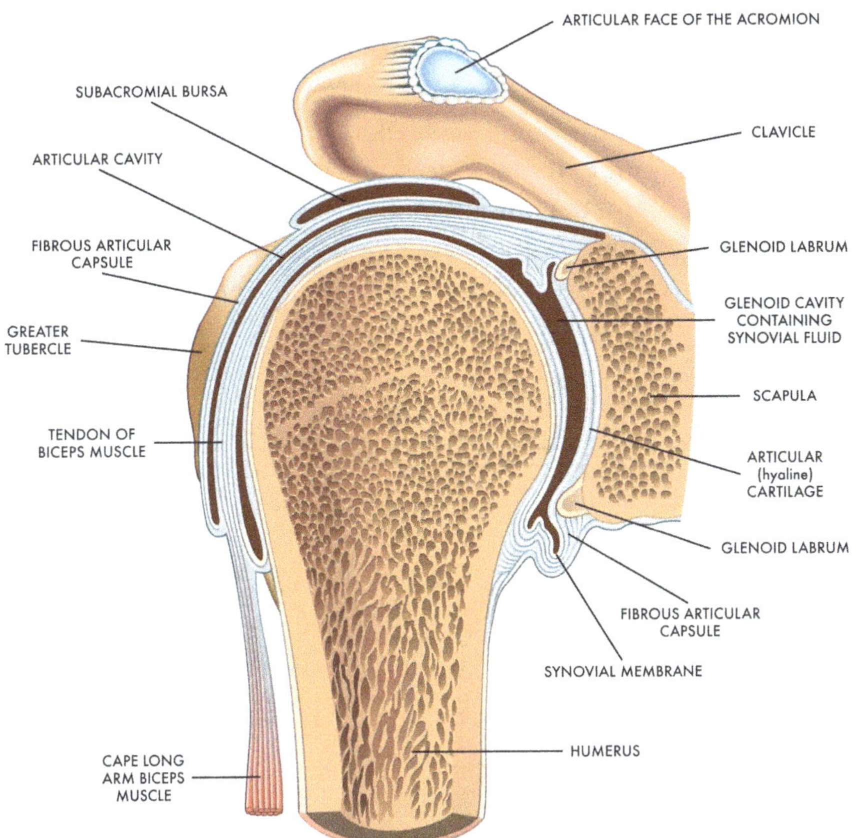

Fig. 1.3.2 Subdeltoid Bursa

1. **Subacromial Bursa**: The fluid-filled sac that reduces friction between the acromion and the rotator cuff tendons.
2. **Subdeltoid Bursa**: The fluid-filled sac located between the deltoid muscle and the shoulder joint capsule. This facilitates smooth motion by allowing the underside of the deltoid muscle to move over the humeral head and capsule.

NERVES

1. **Axillary Nerve**: Innervates the deltoid muscle. This nerve wraps around the humeral neck and on the underside of the deltoid muscle.
2. **Suprascapular Nerve**: Innervates the supraspinatus and infraspinatus muscles and is located on the posterior aspect of the scapula after it travels through the notch of the scapula.

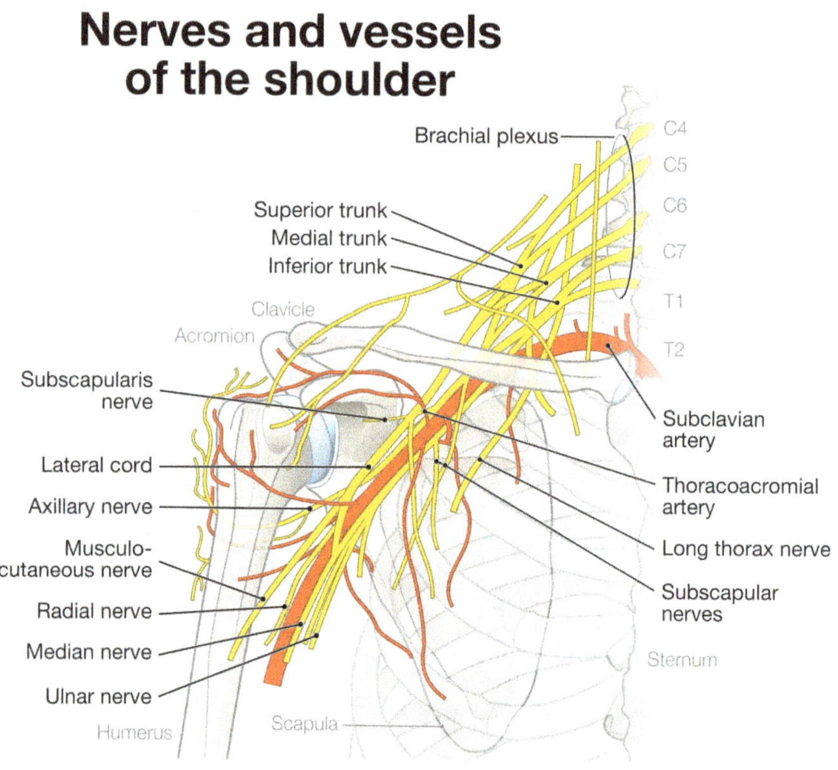

Fig. 1.4 Blood Vessels and Nerves

BLOOD VESSELS

1. **Axillary Artery**: This very important artery that supplies the entire upper extremity travels under the clavicle and is a part of the neurovascular bundle in the axilla (arm pit). It supplies blood to the shoulder as well as to the arm and hand.
2. **Subclavian Artery**: This artery is the portion of the main artery to the arm and hand that is under the clavicle more proximally than the axilla. There are several branches of the Subclavian Artery that supply the shoulder and the chest wall. The artery continues as the axillary artery beyond the clavicle as it enters the arm medial to the humerus.

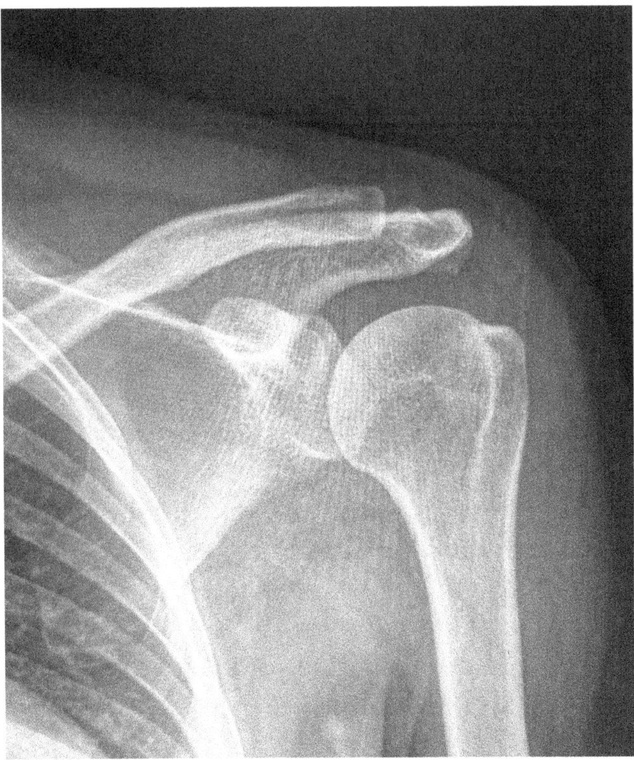

Fig. 1.5 X Ray Shoulder AP and Axillary

LIGAMENTS AND TENDONS:

- **Glenohumeral Ligaments:** Provide stability by reinforcing the joint capsule. The most significant are the superior, middle, and inferior glenohumeral ligaments.
- **Coracohumeral Ligament:** Provides additional stability by connecting the coracoid process of the scapula to the humerus.
- **Rotator Cuff Tendons:** Include the tendons of four muscles (supraspinatus, infraspinatus, teres minor, and subscapularis) that stabilize the shoulder joint and allow for rotation and lifting movements.
- **Biceps Tendon:** The tendon of the long head of the biceps brachii also contributes to shoulder stability as it passes through the bicipital groove of the humerus.

MUSCLES:

- **Rotator Cuff Muscles:** Provide dynamic stability and control of the shoulder joint.
    - **Supraspinatus:** Abduction of the arm.
    - **Infraspinatus and Teres Minor:** External rotation of the arm.
    - **Subscapularis:** Internal rotation of the arm.
- **Deltoid:** Covers the shoulder and is responsible for arm abduction. Moving the arm away from the body.
- **Pectoralis Major and Minor:** Assist in shoulder flexion, adduction, and internal rotation.
- **Latissimus Dorsi:** Involved in shoulder extension, adduction, and internal rotation.
- **Trapezius, Levator Scapulae, and Rhomboids:** Act on the scapula to allow full shoulder motion.

BIOMECHANICS AND PHYSIOLOGY

The shoulder joint, also known as the glenohumeral joint, is one of the most complex and mobile joints in the human body. It allows a wide range of motion in multiple directions, which is essential for various upper limb functions. The trade off for this very hypermobile joint is some risk of instability. The stability of the shoulder is a combination of muscle strength and ligament presence and capsular strength of the glenohumeral shoulder joint.

BIOMECHANICS:

- **Movement:** The shoulder joint allows flexion, extension, abduction, adduction, internal rotation, external rotation, and circumduction. The joint's structure, with a shallow glenoid fossa and a large humeral head, provides extensive mobility at the expense of inherent stability.
- **Stability:** Stability is achieved through a combination of static structures (bones, ligaments, joint capsule) and dynamic structures (muscles, tendons). The rotator cuff muscles play a crucial role in maintaining the humeral head's position within the glenoid cavity, especially during arm movements.
- **Scapulohumeral Rhythm:** Refers to the coordinated movement between the scapula and the humerus during shoulder motion. For every 2 degrees of humeral elevation, there is approximately 1 degree of scapular rotation, allowing for greater range of motion and functional stability.

NERVE SUPPLY:

- The shoulder joint is primarily innervated by the **brachial plexus**, which includes nerves like the **axillary nerve**, **suprascapular nerve**, and **subscapular nerve**. These nerves provide motor (movement) and sensory (feeling) innervation to the shoulder muscles and joints.

VASCULAR SUPPLY:

- Blood supply to the shoulder comes from branches of the **subclavian artery** and **axillary artery**, including the **suprascapular artery**, **circumflex humeral arteries**, and **thoracoacromial artery**.

PATHOPHYSIOLOGY:

- **Instability:** Due to its wide range of motion, the shoulder is prone to dislocations and subluxations (partial), often resulting from trauma or repetitive overhead activities.
- **Rotator Cuff Injuries:** Tears or inflammation of the rotator cuff tendons can lead to pain, weakness, and limited range of motion.
- **Impingement Syndrome:** Occurs when the rotator cuff tendons are compressed during upward and forward shoulder movement, leading to pain and inflammation.
- **Arthritis:** Degenerative changes in the glenohumeral or acromioclavicular joint can lead to pain and stiffness. This pain can vary from 3/10 to 10/10.

The shoulder joint's complex structure and function make it versatile but also susceptible to various injuries and conditions, particularly in athletes or individuals engaged in repetitive overhead activities.

2 ROTATOR CUFF INJURIES AND TREATMENTS

INTRODUCTION

In this chapter I'm going to discuss how to diagnose and treat these specific injuries ranging from the conservative to the surgical options. From the beginning of an assessment of these injuries as an Orthopedic Surgeon, I always include a history, physical examination, any X-rays or lab tests that may be necessary to get an accurate diagnosis before I embark on a treatment plan. I'll also discuss my initial findings and the treatment plan with the patient. I consider the treatments that are the most efficient and safest with the best outcome for my patients in every case. Let's begin.

DESCRIPTION OF INJURY

Injuries to the shoulder may be a single event or could be due to repetitive trauma over time, all affecting the muscles and tendons of the rotator cuff in the shoulder. There are also the effects of aging as well as wear and tear on the rotator cuff that aren't the result of obvious injuries. Oftentimes these injuries and conditions may overlap.

ROTATOR CUFF TEARS

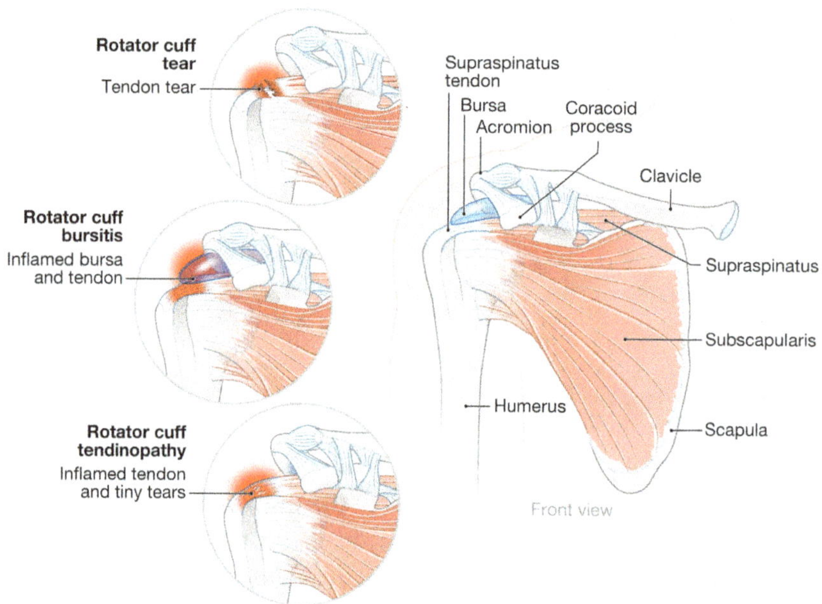

Fig. 2.1.1 Rotator Cuff Tear

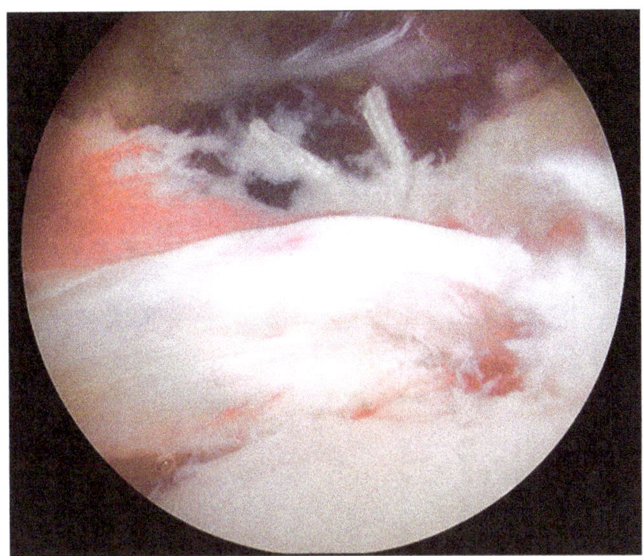

Fig. 2.1.2 Rotator Cuff Tear

Description: Rotator cuff tears occur when the tendons connecting the shoulder muscles to the bone are torn, often due to repetitive stress or a sudden injury. Tears may be very small or very large with all muscles and tendons torn off the greater tuberosity (bump wear tendons attach) of the humerus. Early in the analysis an MRI can easily confirm the size and seriousness of the tear.

Symptoms: There can be pain when lifting or lowering the arm in rotator cuff tears. There may also be pain at rest or in certain positions, such as at night when one is trying to sleep on the side of the shoulder injury or on the opposite side. Reaching forward is usually very painful as well. Pain can range from 0/10 (no pain) to 10 out of 10 (severe pain). Movement of the shoulder with a rotator cuff tear can reach 10/10 pain, but at rest it can be 5/10 to 6/10.

Weakness of the shoulder is very common. This is usually associated with lifting in any direction. Just the weight of the outstretched arm can be very painful with a great deal of weakness. In my experience, the greater the weakness, the larger the tear, especially in the early stages of assessment within approximately three to seven days of the injury. If there is massive weakness within the first day and no ability to lift the arm at all is noted, there is probably a complete massive tear of all the muscle and tendons of the rotator cuff, which can be confirmed by MRI.

Clinical Exam. In order to determine a diagnosis of rotator cuff tear and to assess the severity of the tear I perform a clinical examination. The basics of the exam are to ask the patient to move the arm on their own if they can, but usually pain limits motion of the patient. Also if the tear is large they won't be able to lift their arm in any direction.

During my exam of the patient I palpate, or touch, the muscles involved such as the deltoid and the rotator cuff muscles with a certain pressure that would elicit a certain level of pain. This helps me localize where the muscles are torn. In addition specific areas of tenderness deep in the front of the shoulder joint as well as in the area of the subacromial space indicate specific other diagnoses for me.

Diagnostic Injection Over the many years of my practice I have used anesthetic injection as a diagnostic tool as follows: I inject a solution of Marcaine, Lidocaine, and DepoMedrol (a steroid derivative) early in the case. If the anesthetic numbs up the shoulder and the patient can move the arm in the upward direction, this is very significant. This means that the patient was not moving the shoulder due to pain. If the patient still cannot move the shoulder when it is numbed up, then that is due to a massive tear of the rotator cuff. However, if the patient can move the shoulder upward after the anesthetic injection, this is a better prognosis and the outcome will be better and occur in a shorter time.

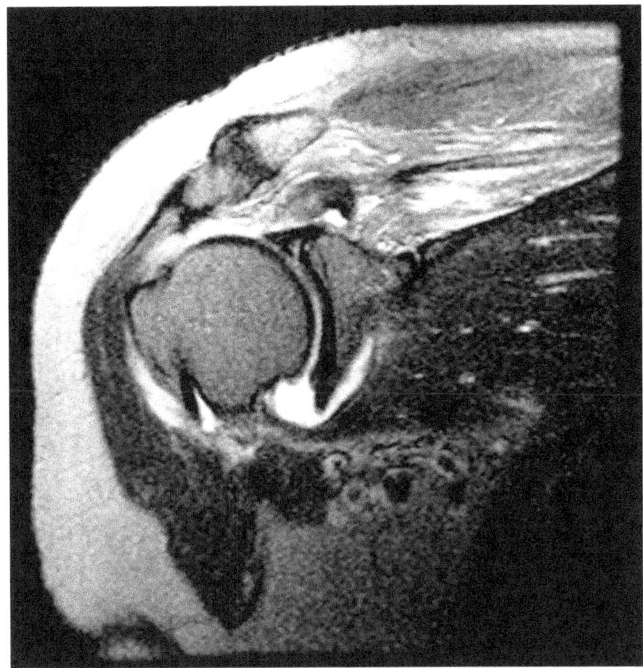

Fig. 2.2 MRI Rotator Cuff Tear Plus A-C Arthritis

Imaging Studies Rotator cuff tears are primarily diagnosed based on clinical examination, but I find that imaging studies like MRI or ultrasound are very important to an accurate diagnosis of rotator cuff tear tear or even loose bodies or bursitis. An MRI of the shoulder demonstrates if there is a tear of the rotator cuff. If there is a large tear with retraction this can also be demonstrated. The MRI can be done with or without a dye Gadolinium that sometimes is used to increase the detail of the image.

Blood Tests These aren't typically used to diagnose a rotator cuff tear directly, however these lab tests may be ordered to rule out other conditions or to assess the overall health of the patient.

Some lab tests that might be considered for general metabolic conditions in the context of shoulder pain or suspected rotator cuff tear include:

1. **Complete Blood Count (CBC):** To check for signs of infection, anemia, or other systemic conditions that might cause or complicate shoulder pain.
2. **C-Reactive Protein (CRP) and Erythrocyte Sedimentation Rate (ESR):** To assess for inflammation or infection, particularly if there is concern about conditions like septic arthritis or other inflammatory diseases.
3. **Rheumatoid Factor (RF) and Anti-Cyclic Citrullinated Peptide (Anti-CCP):** To rule out rheumatoid arthritis if the clinical presentation suggests an inflammatory or autoimmune condition.
4. **Thyroid Function Tests:** Hypothyroidism is sometimes associated with musculoskeletal issues including shoulder pain, and might be considered if there are other clinical indications.

These tests are generally part of a broader diagnostic workup if the clinical picture is unclear or if the patient has other symptoms that suggest a more systemic condition.

MRI imaging and physical examination definitely remain the cornerstone of diagnosing a rotator cuff tear.

DIAGNOSIS

After an extensive workout including the physical examination special studies a diagnosis of rotator cuff tear can be made. My experience is that once an accurate diagnosis is made a plan for treatment is then outlined. I always in the past have treated the patient first conservatively and then if surgery is indicated this is done with full informed consent of the patient. As a physician I always kept in mind "Do No Harm" in treating my patients.

CONSERVATIVE TREATMENT

The first assessment of the shoulder should be the exam for strength, swelling, and pain. Range of motion also needs to be tested initially. After this initial evaluation, if it is an acute injury within 24 to 48 hours, the initial treatment is ice, gentle range of motion, and rest in a sling. Anti-inflammatories should also be started at this time. Examples of these non-steroid anti-inflammatories (NSAIDS) Naprosyn, ibuprofen, Celebrex, and many other over the counter medications that do not require a prescription.

Periodic movement is essential, either done by the patient moving their own shoulder by themself or having someone in the household or a physical therapist move the shoulder with them.

After the first 72 hours, usually heat should help reduce the pain and swelling better than ice. The heat encourages the blood flow to come and remove products of injury as well as excessive tissue fluid.

If the physical examination indicates the patient can actively elevate the arm even slightly, this is a good sign to continue the conservative treatment.

PHYSICAL THERAPY

A physical therapist at this early stage would be extremely beneficial in maintaining the range of motion of the patient's shoulder. The therapist will be able to move the shoulder further than the patient would be able to do on their own. This movement is very gentle but complete and will not only improve range of motion, but also can reduce pain, eventual swelling, and function. Physical therapy three times a week is ideal and it may take several weeks or sometimes months to gain the full range of motion and strength of the shoulder. If there is a small tear, this along with other conservative treatments may suffice to heal the shoulder.

Steroid Injection for Shoulder Injury

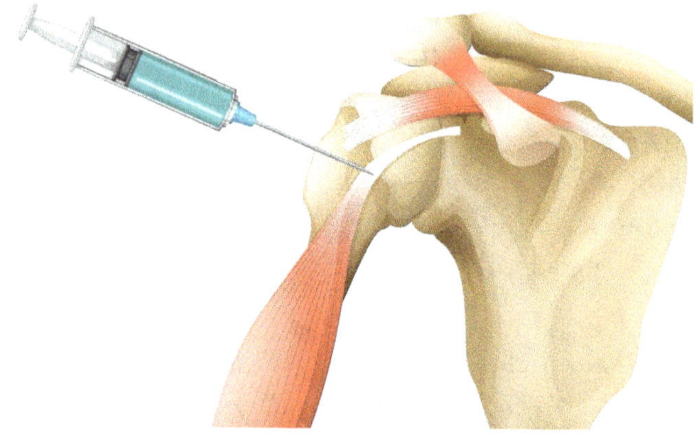

Fig.2.3 Subacromial Steroid Injection

Injections. I also usually use corticosteroid injections mixed with local short and long term anesthetic into the subacromial space. These injections have been used for decades with great benefit. One or two shots may be curative over a period of three to four weeks for small tears. Large tears will not be cured by simple injections and physical therapy. After three months of this treatment, if there is continued weakness, limited range of motion, and pain, then surgery is usually required to correct the problem. An MRI must first be done prior to surgery to confirm and estimate the size of the tear as well as the amount it has retracted.

RISKS OF OVER IMMOBILIZATION

A word of caution. Even though rest is recommended using a sling or a shoulder brace, this should not be done continuously 24/7. Having the shoulder immobilized continuously in this position for weeks or months will lead to stiffness and possibly even a frozen shoulder. It is far better to have a therapist three times per week gently move the shoulder through as much range as possible without hurting the patient too much. If one can maintain the range of motion in this fashion even if a person needs surgical repair, the outcome will be better.

In most cases of rotator cuff tears such as small or even medium size tears, there can be a good outcome with these conservative measures over a two to three month time frame. Usually, if the tears are more trouble, larger, more painful or the shoulder feels loose then consideration for surgical intervention must be made.

SURGICAL TREATMENT

ROTATOR CUFF REPAIR

In most rotator cuff repairs there are several choices. For the last 35 years, arthroscopic surgery has been available, allowing rotator cuff repairs to be done arthroscopically. It is less invasive, the healing is quicker, and the scarring is less. Recent studies have shown that any reoperations that are needed for rotator cuff repairs are less frequent if the surgery is done arthroscopically versus an open procedure. Depending on the training, experience, and skill of the surgeon, arthroscopy is recommended over open procedures unless the tissue condition is poor and special suturing is required.

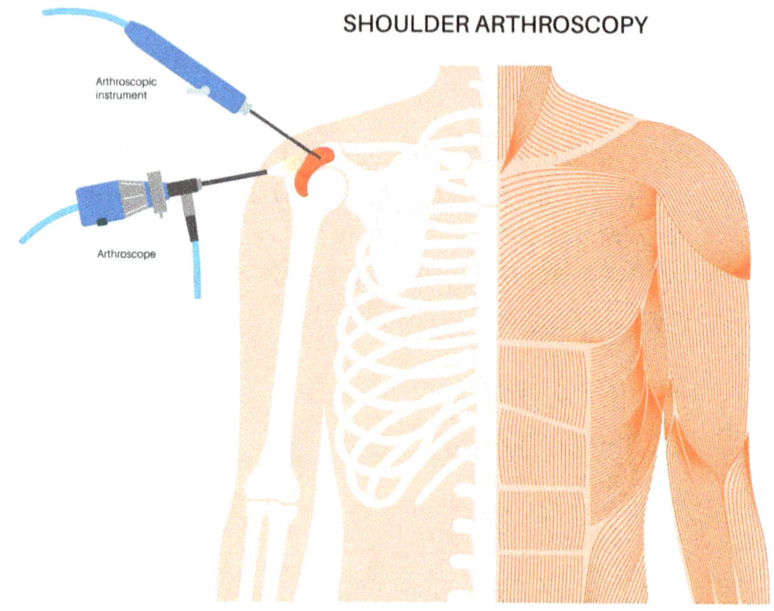

Fig.2.4.1 Arthroscopy Shoulder Setup

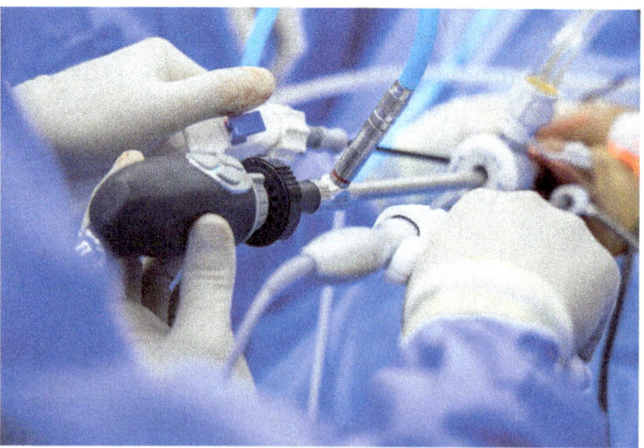

Fig. 2.4.2 Arthroscopy Shoulder Setup

Arthroscopy. This is a technique using a rigid small tube that has fiber optics in it to bring the light inside the joint and a lens to view the inside of the joint. For 46 years I used this technique which utilized a television monitor and very small surgical instruments that are unique to working inside of joints. As it relates to the shoulder, the areas in the joint can be visualized very magnified. In the subacromial space where the rotator cuff is torn, this structure can be visualized very clearly and suturing of a rotator cuff as well as placement of anchors can be accomplished accurately and successfully. **Fig. 2.4.2** Demonstrates an arthroscopic setup including the arthroscope, the fiber optic setup, and the television monitor and patient positioning. Some of the instruments are also displayed.

As one of the first arthroscopists in Southern California,I've been doing arthroscopic surgery since 1978 as a primary portion of my practice and have utilized it hundreds of times in shoulder surgery. The technique is somewhat difficult to learn, especially in the shoulder and skilled training as well as repetitive practice needs to be done by the surgeon before embarking on this procedure in patients.

REOPERATION RATE

In a study by Nircole M Truong et al, in Arthroscopy, Sports Medicine and Rehabilitation volume 3 issue 6 December 2021 they studied 534,076 patients diagnosed with a full thickness rotator cuff tear. Thirty seven percent (37%) of these patients underwent a repair and 73% of these were arthroscopic repairs. Also 27% were open procedures and were more likely to have reoperations 11.3% of the time. The arthroscopic group had reoperations in 9.5% of the time and the patients who are at age 50 to 59 had the greatest rate of reoperation which was 14%. No patient younger than 40 years old had to have reoperation.Their conclusion in this article was arthroscopic surgery in a young person is more beneficial than in an older person. This is probably due to the tissue quality and the lack of arthritis.

STEPS OF AN ARTHROSCOPIC ROTATOR CUFF REPAIR

1. Preoperative Preparation:

- **Medical Evaluation**: The patient undergoes a thorough medical evaluation, including imaging studies (MRI, X-rays) to assess the extent of the rotator cuff tear.
- **Anesthesia**: The patient is given regional anesthesia (nerve block) or general anesthesia, depending on the surgeon's preference and the patient's condition.

2. Patient Positioning:

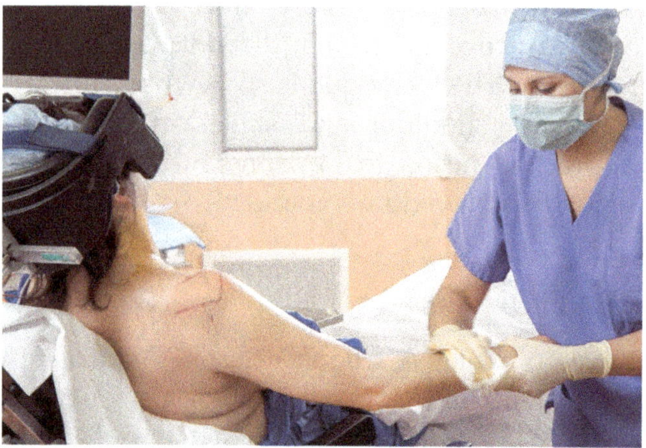

Fig. 2.5 Beach Chair Position

- The patient is positioned either in the beach chair position (semi-upright) or the lateral decubitus position (lying on the side) to allow optimal access to the shoulder. My preference is the beach chair position as everything appears more anatomical to me.

3. Portal Placement:

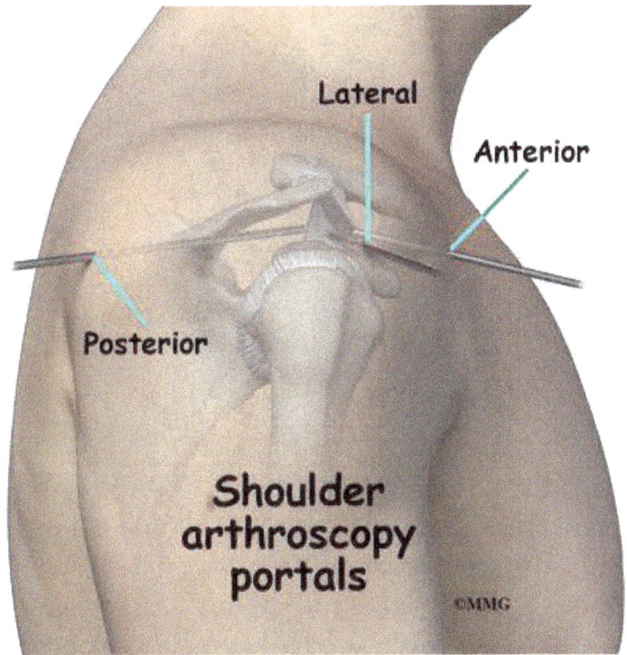

Fig. 2.6 Portal Placement

- Small incisions (portals) are made around the shoulder to insert the arthroscopic instruments. Usually 3 portals are used: the posterior for viewing and the lateral and anterior for operating with very small instruments.
- A camera attached to the back of the arthroscope is inserted through one portal to provide a clear view of the shoulder joint on a monitor.

4. Joint Inspection:

- The surgeon examines the entire shoulder joint, including the rotator cuff tendons, biceps tendon, labrum, and cartilage, to identify any additional issues.

5. Debridement:

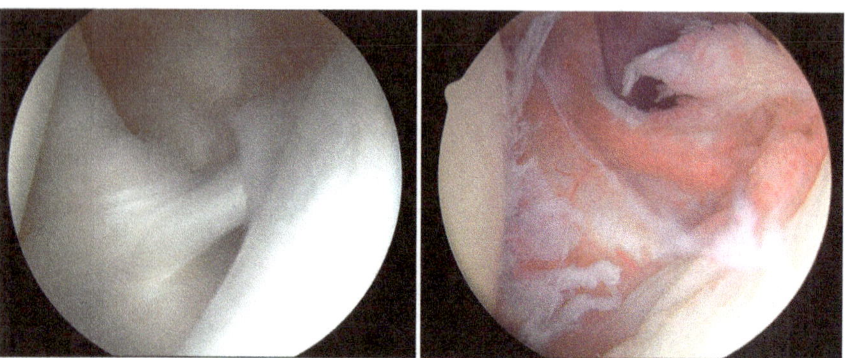

Fig. 2.7 Inspection and Debridement

- Damaged and frayed tissue around the tear is cleaned (debrided) with a motorized shaver blade to create a smooth surface for repair.
- Any bone spurs or other impinging structures are also removed to prevent future irritation. Loose bodies are removed as encountered.

6. Preparation of the Bone:

- The footprint of the rotator cuff tendon on the humerus (upper arm bone) is prepared by removing any remaining soft tissue and roughening the bone surface to promote healing.

7. Anchor Placement:

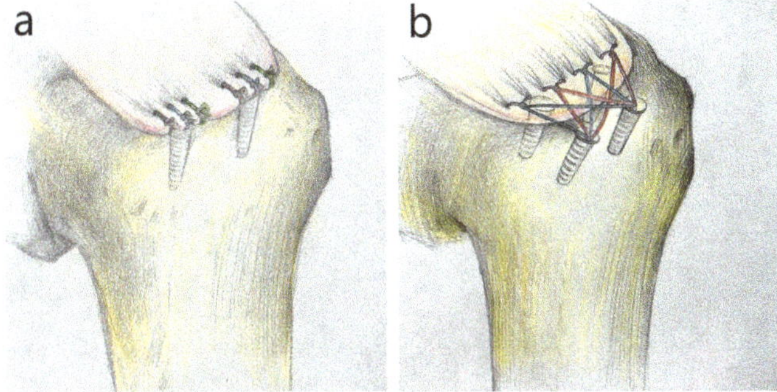

Fig. 2.8 Anchor Placement

- Small anchors, made of metal or bioabsorbable material, are inserted into the bone at the edge of the rotator cuff footprint. These anchors have sutures attached to them.

8. Suturing the Tendon

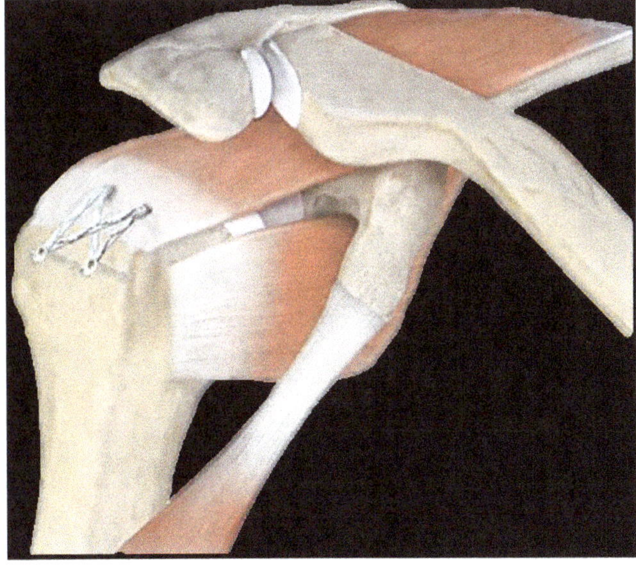

Fig. 2.9.1 Suturing Tendon

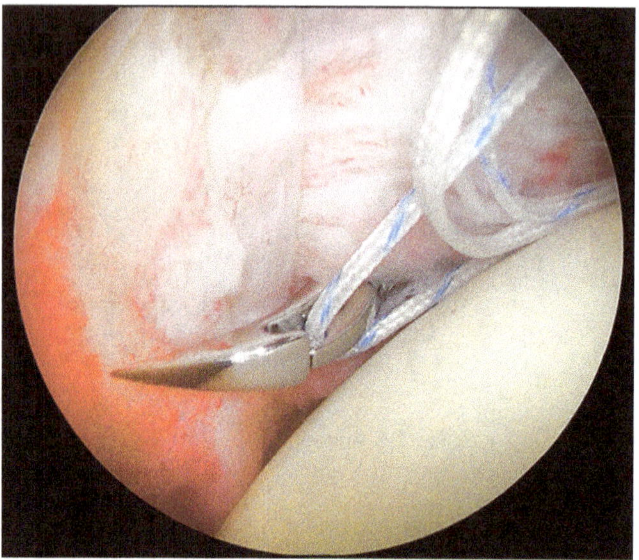

Fig. 2.9.2 Suturing Tendon

The rotator cuff tendons are grasped with specialized instruments.

- The sutures from the anchors are passed through the tendon in a specific pattern to ensure a secure attachment.

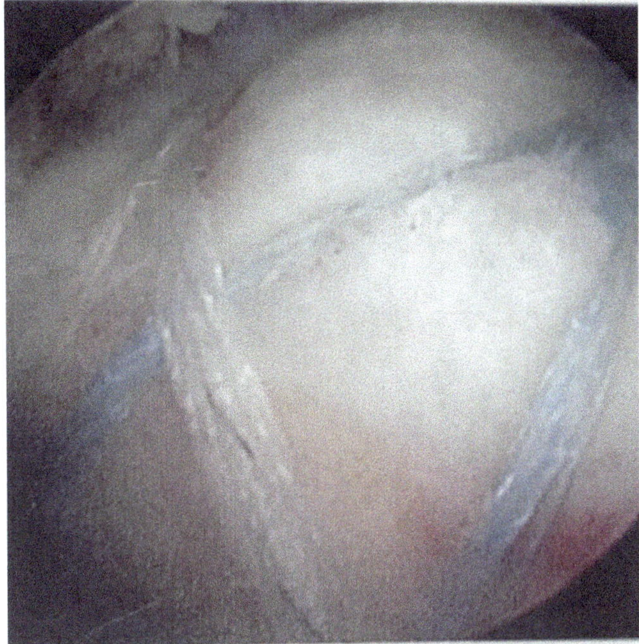

Fig. 2.9.3 Suturing Tendon

- The sutures are tied to pull the tendon back to its original attachment site on the bone.

9. Final Inspection:

- The surgeon inspects the repaired tendon to ensure it is securely attached and properly aligned.
- Any additional repairs (e.g., biceps tendon repair) are performed if necessary.

TYPES OF ANCHORS

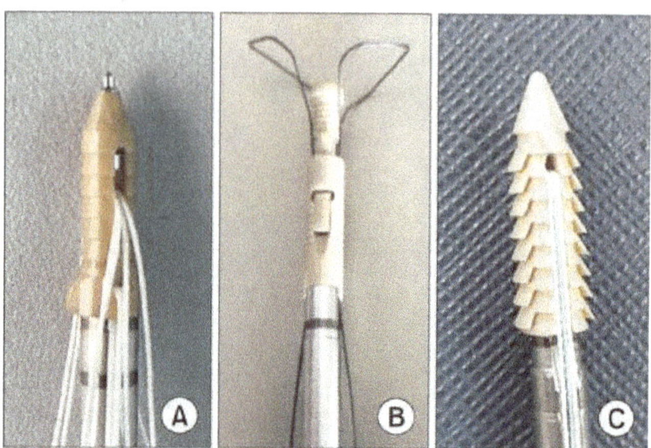

Fig. 2.10 Hybrid Anchors

10. Closure:

- The arthroscopic instruments are removed.
- The small incisions are closed with sutures or surgical tape.
- Sterile dressings are applied to the incision sites.
- A pillow sling is applied.

1. Metal Anchors:

- **Material:** Typically made from titanium or stainless steel.
- **Advantages:**
  - Strong and durable.
  - High visibility on X-rays and other imaging modalities.
- **Disadvantages:**
  - Permanent presence in the body, which can sometimes cause irritation.
  - Potential for interference with MRI.

2. Bioabsorbable Anchors:

- **Material:** Made from polymers that gradually dissolve and are absorbed by the body over time.
- **Advantages:**
    - No long-term foreign material remains in the body.
    - Less risk of long-term irritation or complications.
- **Disadvantages:**
    - Potential for inflammatory reactions as the material degrades.
    - May not be as strong as metal anchors initially.

3. PEEK (Polyether Ether Ketone) Anchors:

- **Material:** A type of biocompatible plastic known for its strength and stability.
- **Advantages:**
    - High biocompatibility with minimal inflammatory response.
    - Radiolucent (does not show up on X-rays), which can be an advantage or disadvantage depending on the clinical situation.
- **Disadvantages:**
    - Permanent presence in the body.
    - Higher cost compared to some other materials.

4. All-Suture Anchors:

- **Material:** Composed entirely of suture material without a solid anchor body.
- **Advantages:**
    - Minimal bone removal required for insertion.
    - Less risk of anchor-related complications.
- **Disadvantages:**
    - May not be suitable for all types of repairs, particularly in poor-quality bone.

○ Limited by the strength of the suture material.

5. Hybrid Anchors

- **Material:** Combine elements of metal and bioabsorbable or PEEK materials.
- **Advantages:**
  ○ Aim to provide a balance of strength and biocompatibility.
  ○ Gradual degradation of the absorbable component while maintaining initial fixation strength.
- **Disadvantages:**
  ○ Complexity in design may lead to higher costs.

FACTORS INFLUENCING ANCHOR SELECTION

- **Type of Repair:** The specific procedure being performed (e.g., rotator cuff repair, labral repair) and the nature of the injury.
- **Bone Quality:** The patient's bone density and quality can affect the choice of anchor, with stronger materials preferred for weaker bones.
- **Surgeon Preference:** Surgeons may have preferences based on their experience and familiarity with specific types of anchors.
- **Patient Factors:** Allergies, sensitivities, and the patient's overall health may influence the choice of materials.
- **Postoperative Imaging:** Considerations for future imaging studies, such as the need to avoid metal artifacts in MRI scans.

Choosing the right type of surgical anchor is crucial for the success of shoulder surgeries. The decision is based on various factors, including the type of injury, patient-specific considerations, and the surgeon's expertise. Each type of anchor has its advantages and potential drawbacks, and the choice should be made collaboratively between the surgeon and patient to ensure the best possible outcome.

3 SHOULDER DISLOCATION AND SUBLUXATION

Shoulder dislocation happens when the humeral head pops out of the glenoid cup or shoulder socket, and this is commonly due to a fall or direct blow. This popping out can be anterior, which is the most common, posterior or inferior.

This is an orthopedic emergency because pressure on the axillary artery occurs when the shoulder is dislocated in this fashion.

The partial sliding of the humeral head out of the glenoid cup is called subluxation. Subluxation can be an annoyance, but by itself is not an emergency. After repetitive subluxations with pain it may be serious enough to perform surgery similar to that for a shoulder dislocation.

Shoulder dislocation

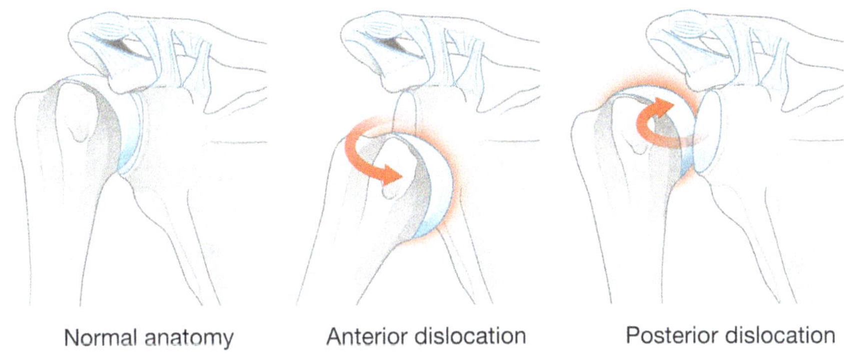

Fig. 3.1 Anterior Shoulder Dislocation

Symptoms: This injury is extremely painful 10/10, especially if occurring for the first time. The patient has an immobilized shoulder joint in various positions, usually down and forward. There is some swelling and bruising, but this usually occurs later. There is numbness or tingling of the hand immediately.

Clinical Exam. When I examine a patient for dislocation it's usually in the office or the emergency room and the position of the arm is fixed usually in a downward inward position that's very painful 10/10 and there may even be some circulatory problem and numbness of the hand and forearm. For an experienced orthopedist such as myself it is an obvious diagnosis and must be addressed quickly. If this is the first time it is dislocated it is a much more painful and difficult situation to correct than someone that has had recurrent dislocations.

DIAGNOSIS

The clinical evaluation supplemented by X-ray MRI and the history leads in most cases to a diagnosis of recurrent subluxation or dislocation. now that a diagnosis is made we can proceed with the treatment of the condition.

TREATMENT

Conservative First dislocations are the most painful 10/10 and dangerous and have to be acted on immediately. Recurrent dislocations may occur with less acute symptoms but still have to be relocated promptly. The treatment of an acutely dislocated shoulder needs to be quick because the circulation to the arm is compromised. The axillary artery is usually pinched because of the displacement of the humeral head out of the glenoid fossa. If circulation is cut off to the arm and hand too long, there are permanent consequences. Therefore, quick action must be taken. Using the standard method of traction with the arm out to the side a sheet is wrapped around the chest pulled by another provider. The surgeon grasping the forearm and hand with steady traction (and mild sedation) the humeral will pop back into the glenoid. This is putting the ball back into the socket. X-rays must be taken after this procedure to make sure there were no fractures caused.

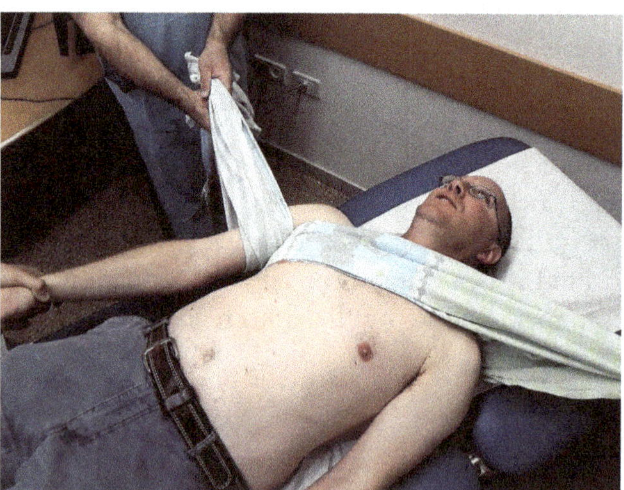

Fig. 3.2 Reducing a Shoulder

Usually, the humeral head will pop back into the glenoid. Most of the time, a sedative is required to relax the patient and the muscles. Occasionally, a general anesthetic is required. as illustrated above two persons are usually required to relocate the humeral head one is stabilizing the chest and trunk the other is pulling on the arm laterally this is a standard technique used in emergency rooms or in the office. Other options for reducing an anterior dislocation are to pull and internally rotate the humeral ahead into place. This is called the Kocker maneuver.

In most cases of first-time dislocation, the patient does not need surgery. After the shoulder has been put back in place, a sling is applied and pain medication is given. The patient is left in a sling for three to four weeks so the anterior capsule can heal. Then gentle motion is begun. The process to gain full motion back is usually approximately 6 to 8 weeks.

In cases of recurrent dislocation (where someone has frequent dislocations of the shoulder), a non-medical person who is familiar with sports injuries can manipulate the arm back into place at the sports field or the ice rink where the dislocation occurs.

Physical therapy. After the shoulder is put back in place it should be held usually for 6 to 8 weeks some surgeons prefer to only hold it for three to four weeks. Once the surgeon feels that the repair is complete and the healing is complete then physical therapy is needed. Physical therapy is involving gentle range of motion by a physical therapist and strengthening and eventually the patient over a period of several weeks, sometimes months will regain the full range of motion and strength of the shoulder and arm. A therapist might use light weights, Theraband, and manual manipulation to assist in the range of motion and strengthening I believe patient.

Surgical treatment. In most cases of first-time dislocation, the patient does not need surgery. However, in cases where the very young athletic person has an initial dislocation from trauma, I would anticipate that there would be repeat future dislocations and that the patient should consider surgery after the first dislocation.

There have been studies over the years in some European countries, in which early stabilization with a staple in the glenoid has been done after a first dislocation in miners who suffered a high rate of first dislocations. This situation is unusual in the United States.

What is more usual in the U.S. is that after several dislocations, a person needs to have surgery. Depending on the experience of the orthopedic surgeon, an arthroscopic placement of a staple or screw in the anterior glenoid bone can be done by the surgeon. Prior to arthroscopic surgery, this procedure would be done openly through an approximately 4-inch incision, and this gave satisfactory results as well. There are surgeons who are more comfortable with this open procedure today. The results of the surgery can be good to excellent either way it is done.

Here is a general overview of the steps involved in an arthroscopic Bankart repair bony rim.

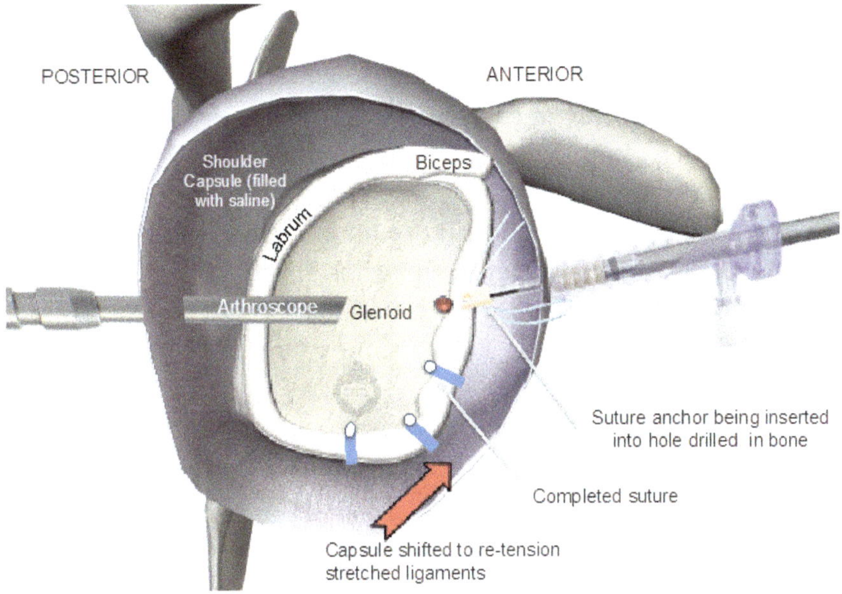

Fig. 3.3 Bankart Repair of Labrum

FOR RECURRENT DISLOCATIONS

BANKART SHOULDER REPAIR (ARTHROSCOPIC) - SURGICAL PROCEDURE AND PREPARATION

Preoperative Preparation:

1. **Patient Evaluation:**
   - Detailed history and physical examination.
   - Imaging: MRI or CT scan to assess the extent of labral tear and associated injuries (e.g., bony Bankart, Hill-Sachs lesion).
   - Discuss risks, benefits, and post-operative rehabilitation with the patient.

2. **Anesthesia:**
   - General anesthesia with regional block (interscalene) is commonly used.
3. **Patient Positioning:**
   - Beach chair or lateral decubitus position, depending on surgeon preference.
   - Ensure proper padding of bony prominences and secure the head and upper body.
4. **Preparation of the Operative Field:**
   - Sterile preparation and draping of the shoulder, arm, and axilla.
   - The arm can move freely or be held in traction. This is determined by the surgeon's preference.

Surgical Procedure:

1. **Portal Placement:**
   - **Posterior Portal:** Main viewing portal, placed 2-3 cm inferior and medial to the posterolateral corner of the acromion.
   - **Anterior Superior Portal:** Through the rotator interval for instrumentation.
   - **Anterior Inferior Portal:** Just above the subscapularis tendon for direct access to the anteroinferior labrum.
2. **Diagnostic Arthroscopy:**
   - A systematic evaluation of the glenohumeral joint is performed, including inspection of the labrum, capsule, biceps tendon, rotator cuff, and articular surfaces.
3. **Preparation of the Glenoid Rim:**
   - The glenoid rim is debrided using a shaver or burr to create a bleeding bony surface for better healing.
   - Any loose or frayed labral tissue is debrided, leaving enough healthy labrum for reattachment.
4. **Anchor Placement:**

- Typically, 3-4 suture anchors are placed along the anterior-inferior glenoid rim.
- Anchors are spaced 1 cm apart from the 5 o'clock to 3 o'clock positions (right shoulder).
- Use a drill guide to insert the anchors, ensuring they are securely seated in the bone.

5. **Labral Repair:**
   - Pass the sutures from the anchors through the labrum using a suture-passing device.
   - A simple mattress or knotless suture technique may be used depending on the surgeon's preference.
   - The labrum is securely reattached to the glenoid rim, ensuring anatomic restoration of the capsulolabral complex.

6. **Capsular Shift (if necessary):**
   - If there is capsular redundancy or instability, a capsular shift may be performed by advancing the capsule superiorly.

7. **Closure:**
   - The portals are closed with sutures.
   - The joint is thoroughly irrigated to remove any loose debris.

8. **Postoperative Dressing and Immobilization:**
   - Sterile dressings are applied.
   - The shoulder is typically placed in a sling with the arm in slight abduction and internal rotation.

Postoperative Care:

1. **Pain Management:**
   - Regional block combined with oral analgesics.
   - Anti-inflammatory medications as needed.

2. **Rehabilitation:**
   - **Phase 1 (0-4 weeks):** Immobilization with limited passive range of motion exercises.

- **Phase 2 (4-8 weeks):** Gradual increase in range of motion, avoiding excessive external rotation.
- **Phase 3 (8-12 weeks):** Strengthening exercises focusing on the rotator cuff and scapular stabilizers.
- **Phase 4 (3-6 months):** Return to sport-specific activities and gradual return to full activity.

3. **Follow-Up:**
   - Regular follow-up visits to monitor progress and adjust the rehabilitation protocol as needed.
   - Imaging may be used to assess the healing and position of the repair.

4 SHOULDER IMPINGEMENT AND BICEPS TENDINITIS

SHOULDER IMPINGEMENT OCCURS WHEN THE ROTATOR CUFF tendons and bursae are pinched during upward shoulder movements, which is usually due to repetitive overhead activities. Forward position is also a very common position for impingement of the shoulder.

Symptoms. Sharp pain when lifting the arm forward or sidewise. Due to pain, there is also weakness of the muscles, and lifting is difficult, especially moving forward and to the side. There is a limited range of motion also due to pain and gradual tightness of the tissues from protecting the shoulder from pain. Without movement throughout the full range of motion due to pain, scarring occurs in the joint, and as the scarring progresses, the joint gets tighter, and movement gets more painful and more restricted.

Treatment. Non-surgical treatment. Initially rest. Then, gradually physical therapy focuses on stretching and strengthening. The goal at this early stage is to maintain a range of motion as close to full as possible without hurting the patient too much while they're awake.

Anti-inflammatory medication orally is required to reduce inflammation. Ice is helpful after a therapy session. Corticosteroid injections, along with short-acting (1-2 hr.) and long (12-14 hr.) acting anesthetics, are very beneficial to eliminating severe pain during range of motion therapy. The injection is put in the subacromial space where the inflammation is occurring. It may take several of these injections over a period of a year to permanently eliminate the problem and avoid surgery.

Physical therapy. Physical therapy is extremely important in the recovery of the range of motion and strength in this type of condition. An experienced therapist will use passive range of motion, stretching, and light weights, and Theraband all with the purpose of improving the strength and range of motion of the shoulder. depending on the patient's tolerance for pain and the degree of scarring and inflammation in the shoulder physical therapy may take between six weeks and up to six months to reach maximum benefit. The patient may even require pain pills during this physical therapy period to get a better benefit out of the sessions.

Surgical. When conservative methods fail to achieve a relatively full range of motion without pain, then it is appropriate to recommend surgical intervention.

Under general anesthesia, the arm is manipulated throughout a full range of motion with audible and palpable crunching and popping. This sound is the breaking up of scar tissue in the shoulder. This is a necessary first step, and even though a full range of motion is achieved, surgery is now done to remove the excess scar tissue, cauterize bleeding, and, in most cases, remove some bone from the anterior edge of the acromion and the lateral edge of the acromion as well as thin the bone.

Surgical decompression of the subacromial space by removing bone with a burr from the anterior, lateral, and inferior portions of the acromion is frequently done. General anesthesia is always required.

This surgical procedure, now always done arthroscopically under direct vision, is very successful when needed. Usually, three small punctures are required and only one small stitch in each of the punctures is done. The shoulder is iced for two to three days after the procedure and movement is started within hours. Thereafter, my patients usually work with a physical therapist three days a week until most of the full range of motion is achieved. Rarely are there any complications from surgery during this procedure. The following is the breakdown of the surgical procedure of arthroscopic subacromial decompression in detail.

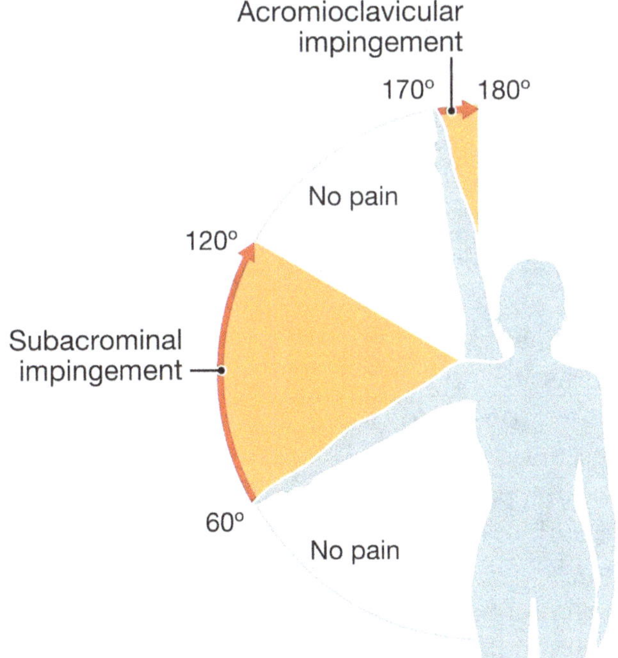

FIG. 4.1 Painful Arc Impingement Test

Arthroscopic Subacromial Decompression (ASD) is a minimally invasive surgical procedure used to treat shoulder impingement syndrome, a condition where the rotator cuff tendons become irritated or compressed as they pass through the subacromial space, the area between the acromion (a bony projection on the scapula) and the rotator cuff.

1. **Anesthesia:** The patient is usually placed under general anesthesia or regional anesthesia (e.g., a nerve block) to ensure they are pain-free during the procedure. Under general anesthesia, the patient must be intubated while asleep.
2. **Patient Positioning:**
   - My patients are typically placed in the beach chair position, basically sitting in a reclined position. Most of the procedures I have done used a general anesthetic.
3. **Arthroscopic Access:**
   - Three small incisions (portals) are made around the shoulder to allow the insertion of the arthroscope attached to a small camera. In the other two portals, surgical instruments are inserted. The posterior portal is used for viewing, whereas the anterior portal and lateral portals are used for operating using various small arthroscopic instruments. One instrument is a burr that also sucks particles of bone and tissue. Another is a grasper to hold tissue and remove loose bodies. The arthroscope provides a magnified view of the shoulder joint on a large TV monitor. So, with everything so magnified, it is very difficult to miss any pathology or problem in my experience.
4. **Subacromial Space Inspection:**
   - inflammation, bony spurs, or other abnormalities contributing to impingement.

Calcific tendinitis and bursitis

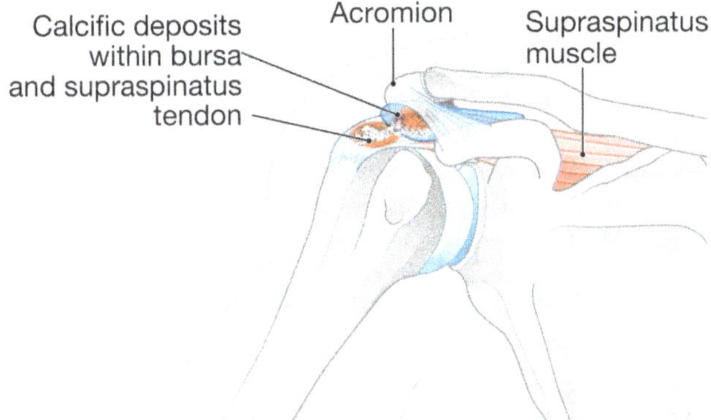

Fig. 4.2 Calcific Tendonitis

- The rotator cuff tendons, the bursa (a fluid-filled sac), and the acromion are closely inspected. Calcium deposits are often encountered and are removed **at this time.**

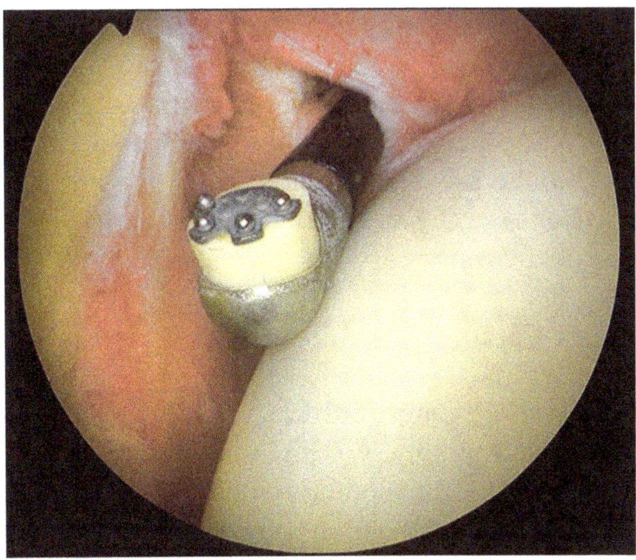

Fig. 4.3 Arthroscopic Subacromial Decompression

5. **Decompression:**
   - **Bursal Debridement:** The inflamed bursa is removed to create more space in the subacromial area. All the raw soft tissue is cauterized to prevent bleeding and recurrence.
   - **Acromioplasty:** The undersurface of the acromion is reshaped to remove any bone spurs or irregularities that might be causing impingement. This is usually done with a burr, a rotating surgical tool that grinds away the bone as it vacuums away the bony debris.
   - **Coracoacromial Ligament Release:** In most of my cases, the coracoacromial ligament is partially released or removed if it is contributing to the impingement. In my cases, this is always done using an electrocautery cutting knife.
6. **Final Inspection:**
   - After decompression, the surgeon rechecks the subacromial space to ensure adequate clearance for the rotator cuff tendons and smooth movement of the shoulder joint.
7. **Closure:**
   - The arthroscope and instruments are removed, and the joint is irrigated vigorously with an antibiotic solution to prevent infection. Then, the small incisions are closed with sutures or sterile strips. A sterile dressing is applied to the shoulder.

Postoperative Care:

- **Recovery and Rehabilitation:**
  - Postoperative care typically involves physical therapy to restore shoulder motion and strength. The patient may need to wear a sling initially to protect the shoulder but can usually start gentle exercises soon after surgery. This is highly encouraged.

- o Full recovery can take several weeks to months, depending on the severity of the impingement and the individual's response to therapy and pain tolerance during therapy.
- **Outcome:**
  - o Most patients experience significant pain relief and improved shoulder function after ASD. However, the success of the surgery also depends on factors like the extent of any rotator cuff damage and the patient's adherence to rehabilitation protocols.

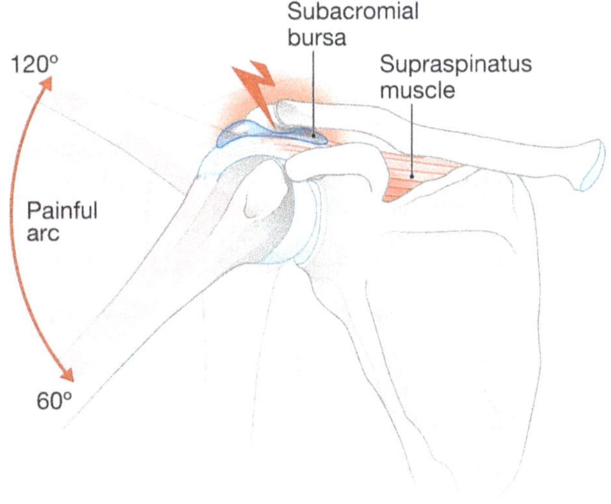

Fig. 4.4 Subacromial Bursitis

BURSITIS

Bursitis is the inflammation of the bursa, the fluid-filled sac that reduces friction in the shoulder between the acromion and the humeral head. The bursitis is caused by a pinching of this bursal sack from repetitive motion and occasionally direct trauma. The thickness of the bursa is a great deal of the problem, and this is associated with inflammation that is very painful, especially with movement. This is similar to a condition called impingement syndrome and they usually go together.

Symptoms. There is significant shoulder pain, especially when moving the arm in a forward, lateral, and rotational direction, even when reaching behind into the back area. It's painful. There is associated swelling, and also, on examination, there is tenderness in the anterior and subacromial area of the shoulder joint.

DIAGNOSIS

Once this diagnosis of Bursitis is made with impingement a treatment plan can be made. We plan the outcome to be as efficient and accurate as possible starting with the conservative methods.

Conservative treatment. When symptoms of pain suggest bursitis, anti-inflammatory pills should be utilized from the beginning. Physical physical therapy can improve the patient as well. My favorite and most successful treatment for bursitis is a mixture of corticosteroids, lidocaine, and Marcaine directly into the bursa. Injections are done up to three occasions spaced 2 weeks apart. This should be curative. If the patient does not respond and does not gain an excellent range of motion or loss of pain, then surgery is probably indicated in my opinion.

Physical therapy. The requirement of physical therapy cannot be emphasized enough in early treatment of Bursitis. Once the pain is taken away with injections and oral pain medication a physical therapist should treat the patient three times a week if possible to improve the range of motion and strength of the shoulder. A Physical Therapist would utilize passive range of motion stretching light weights and Theraband and occasionally ultrasound to achieve the goal. And the goal is full range of painless motion.

SURGERY

Anesthesia. For this procedure, general anesthesia is usually required, although in a stoic patient, I have done this under brachial block. The beach chair position is also my preferred method of doing this surgery.

Surgical Treatment of bursitis is similar to treatment for impingement using arthroscopic techniques. Usually, no bony removal is necessary when surgically removing a bursa. The bursa is removed from the subacromial and subdeltoid area when it is found to be thickened and inflamed. This is done with an electrocautery as well as a mechanical shaver, and it is especially important to cauterize any bleeders that are encountered during this process.

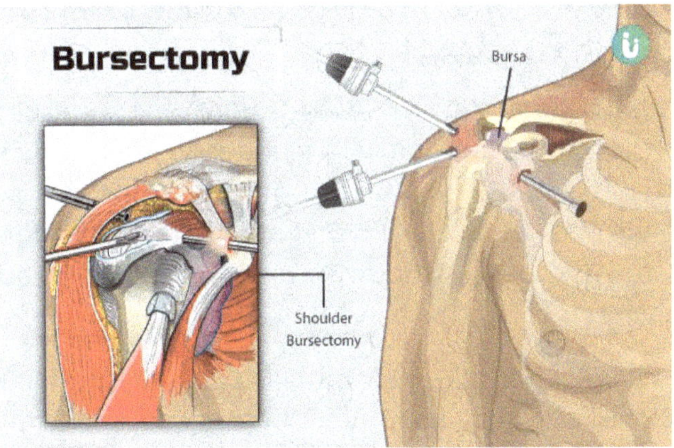

Fig. 4.5 Subacromial Bursectomy

Also associated with this, frequently in older patients, I have found there is some excessive bone from the underside of the acromion, as well as anterior and lateral acromion occasionally.

This bone and spurs are removed to give more room in the subacromial space.

For this procedure, 3 punctures are usually required in the skin, just like in other shoulder arthroscopies.

Postoperative. Bandages, ice, and sling are applied for approximately three to five days. Then gentle motion is started by the physical therapist. These exercises are done two to three days per week until full range of motion is achieved. Oral anti-inflammatory medicine, as well as pain medication, is normally used. A full recovery is anticipated with this surgical procedure of bursectomy and decompression.

The treatment and recovery of bursitis with bursectomy alone is much easier than if it is done with a decompression of bone. Physical therapy proceeds much easier, and the pain is much less.

BICEPS TENDONITIS AND LONG HEAD OF THE BICEPS (LHB) RUPTURE

Biceps tendonitis associated with possible rupture of the long head of the biceps tendon is a condition that can mimic an impingement syndrome. Initially anterior shoulder pain with forward movement is typical. Pain with palpation of the anterior portion of the shoulder over the biceps tendon long head is also typical of this condition

Patient History: in this condition there is a sudden onset of pain in the anterior shoulder with a popping or tearing sensation. The patient can accurately locate where the pain was at the time of the rupture of the long head of the biceps tendon. Also the patient reports weakness of the arm especially in flexion.

Symptoms and History. The patient usually presents with a history of several months of pain in the anterior aspect of the shoulder that is worsened by movement. The patient reports increasing pain with lifting of any object elevated above horizontal. Also they report occasional snapping of the shoulder and they can pinpoint with their finger the area of pain anteriorly. Also some patients that present after several months of pain have other muscles weakened.

Physical Examination: On the many thousands of exams I have performed over my 43 years there is a pattern that has several elements to it. There is tenderness over the bicipital groove. There is also pain when the patient resists forward flexion of the shoulder in which the elbow is flexed and the forearm against resistance is supinated (palm upward). This is referred to as the Speed's Test.

A similar test is the Yergason's Test. In this the patient feels pain or tenderness in the bicipital grove when the patient supinates the forearm against resistance while the elbow is flexed at 90°.

If the biceps tendon is ruptured there may be a **Popeye sign** that is a bulge in the lower arm from the biceps muscle.

When I examine a patient that has reported the symptoms of a sudden pop or tearing sensation in the right shoulder associated with pain I look for the defect in the upper arm of the biceps tendon the muscle has gone down to the distal end and it is demonstrated as a Popeye deformity period

There is often bruising in the arm also called ecchymosis and profound weakness of the biceps muscle.

IMAGING

MRI is helpful in assessing the extent of tendon inflammation and ruling out associated shoulder pathologies, like rotator cuff tears or SLAP lesions.

Ultrasound can visualize tendon inflammation, thickening, or partial tears and is also helpful in some cases.

Xray is also very helpful in ruling out fractures or pathology such as arthritis, calcification, or loose bodies.

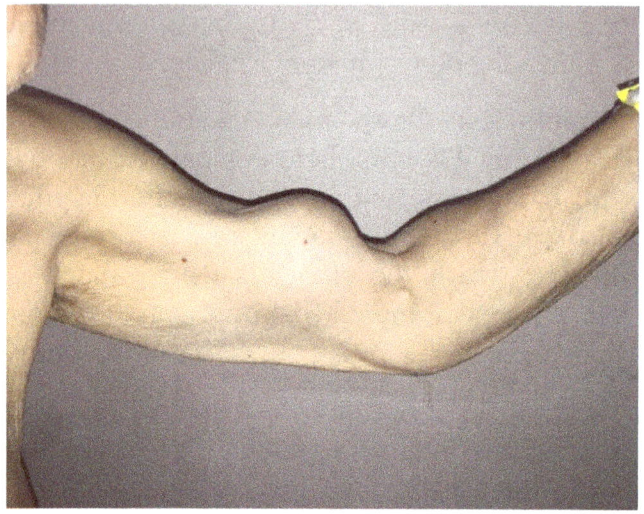

Fig. 4.6 Biceps LH Rupture Popeye Deformity

Imaging. Ultrasound can confirm the diagnosis by showing retraction of the tendon.**MRI** can be used to evaluate the rupture and check for associated injuries (e.g., rotator cuff tear).

DIAGNOSIS

Now that we have an accurate diagnosis of biceps tendonitis or rupture of the biceps tendon we can proceed with treatment. The treatment needs to be safe, efficient and accurate. We start with the conservative and least invasive and then progress to either an arthroscopic tenodesis or tenotomy as we describe below

TREATMENT OF BICEPS TENDONITIS

CONSERVATIVE MANAGEMENT: OLDER PATIENTS

Rest. Avoid activities that exacerbate symptoms. **Ice.** Apply ice to the affected area to reduce inflammation. **NSAIDs** Use nonsteroidal anti-inflammatory drugs to manage pain and inflammation.

Physical Therapy. Focus on strengthening and stretching the rotator cuff and shoulder girdle muscles and correcting biomechanics.

Injections. Corticosteroid Injections may be considered in cases of persistent inflammation. I use these judiciously and usually limit the injections to three in a six month period. The injections include the corticosteroids to reduce inflammation, lidocaine for short acting anesthetic and Marcaine for long acting anesthetic. This mixture makes it easier on the patient to not have pain from the injection.

SURGICAL TREATMENT IN YOUNGER ATHLETES

- **Indications:** Persistent symptoms despite conservative treatment or if there is an associated pathology (e.g., rotator cuff tear).
- **Options:**
  - **Tenotomy:** Releasing the tendon from its attachment, leading to a "Popeye" deformity.
  - **Tenodesis:** Reattaching the tendon to the humerus, usually in younger, more active patients, to preserve the contour and strength of the muscle.

LHB Rupture

1. Conservative Management:

- **Rest:** Especially if the patient is elderly or not engaged in heavy lifting or overhead activities.
- **Physical Therapy:** Focus on maintaining shoulder range of motion and strengthening surrounding muscles.
- **Pain Management:** NSAIDs or other analgesics.

2. Surgical Treatment:

- **Indications:** Younger patients, high-level athletes, or those requiring significant use of the affected arm.
- **Surgical Options:**

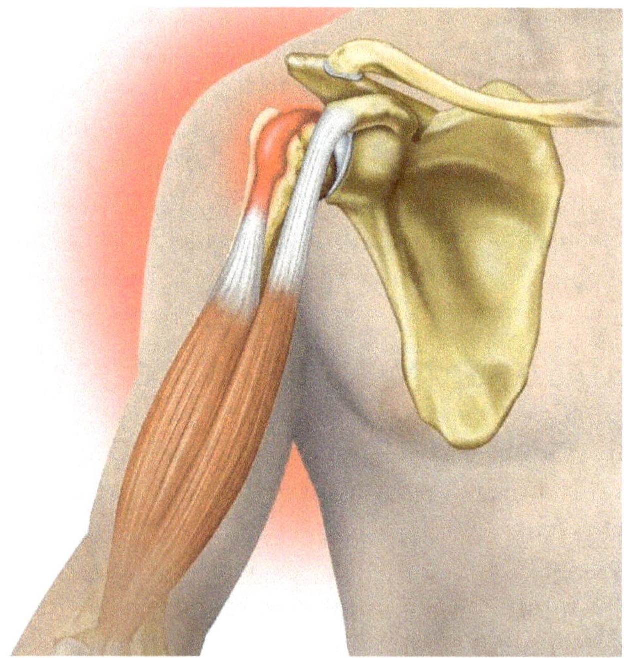

Fig. 4.7 Biceps Tenodesis

- **Tenodesis:** Reattaching the tendon to the humerus in the groove proximally. This can be performed either arthroscopically or as an open procedure.

- ○ **Tenotomy:** Considered in older or less active patients who do not mind a cosmetic deformity and can tolerate a potential decrease in supination strength.

3. Postoperative Physical Therapy

- **Early Phase** The focus is on pain management and gentle range of motion exercises.
- **Strengthening Phase: There is a** gradual introduction of strengthening exercises, particularly for the rotator cuff and biceps, depending on the procedure performed.
- **Return to Activity:** Progressive return to normal activities, typically around 3-6 months postoperatively. Working with a physical therapist shortly after the procedure and extremely helpful. This is a much safer and more efficient way to recover in my experience. A good physical therapist is an essential part of the team for success.

5 LABRAL TEARS

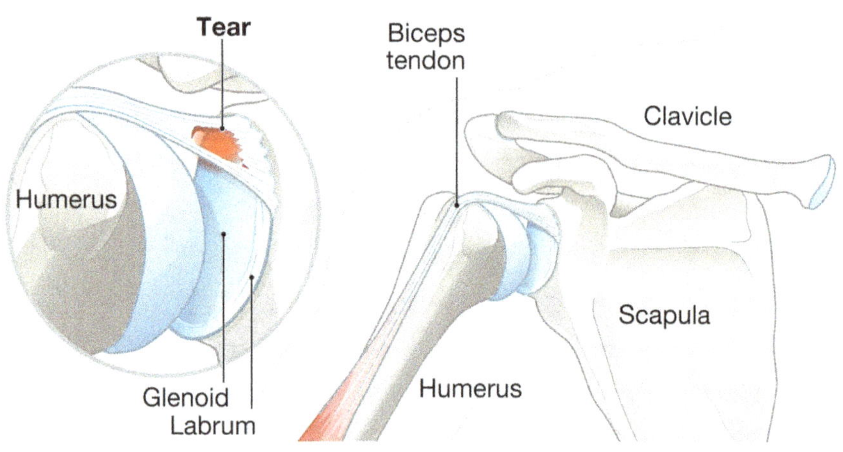

FIG. 5.1 SLAP TEAR

A SLAP (Superior Labrum Anterior and Posterior) lesion refers to an injury to the labrum, the ring of cartilage that surrounds the socket of the shoulder joint. This is due to either a single event but, more often, repetitive trauma from a sports type of injury such as pitching in baseball or throwing in football.

Symptoms. There is often deep shoulder pain and the sensation of catching, locking, or grinding with arm movement. There is also a decrease in the range of motion usually in the upward and slightly forward position. The examiner can often palpate or feel deep in the shoulder joint area. The pain sensation with the labral tear is in a different location than if a patient had bursitis or an impingement syndrome. In the latter situation, the pain is at the most lateral point of the acromion or point of the shoulder. Elevation of the shoulder causes pain in that outer lateral area. Often, a labral tear is difficult to diagnose, and an MRI study is medically necessary. Often a dye called Gadolinium is used to better outline a tear of the labrum.

Imaging. MRI is extremely useful in diagnosing the SLAP lesion. The **MRI** can pick up any other pathologies such as rotator cuff tear, loose bodies, or arthritis. **Ultrasound** can be used in some cases to assess inflammation also..

DIAGNOSIS

Now that we have an accurate diagnosis of a **SLAP lesion** we can proceed with a safe effective efficient treatment that will hopefully totally resolve the problem. We start out with a conservative approach 1st and less invasive approach and then if this does not solve the problem then surgical intervention is required in my opinion.

TREATMENT

Treatment options vary depending on the severity of the lesion, the patient's age, activity level, and symptoms. Here are some common approaches:

CONSERVATIVE MANAGEMENT

Rest and Activity Modification: Reducing activities that aggravate the shoulder, such as overhead movements, heavy lifting, or throwing'

MEDICATION

Medications. I frequently use nonsteroidal anti-inflammatory drugs (NSAIDs) that can help reduce pain and inflammation. Oral anti-inflammatory medication usually takes care of the pain if the pain is not severe. Nsaids usually suffice, but occasionally a stronger pain medication might be required.

Injections. Corticosteroid injections are helpful in a mixture of lidocaine, a short acting anesthetic, and Marcaine a long acting anesthetic. These might be given three times in three months. These injections could relieve symptoms from a small SLAP lesion that does not require surgery.

Physical Therapy focuses on strengthening the rotator cuff muscles and stabilizing the scapula and humeral head in the glenoid fossa. Exercises to improve range of motion and flexibility are also included. Small weights and Theraband are used to help strengthen the shoulder muscles.

SURGERY FOR LABRAL TEAR

When conservative measures fail to resolve the problem by eliminating the pain, catching, or clicking, then I make a surgical recommendation. In my experience, there are patients who have been undiagnosed by previous doctors, and the patient is very frustrated. At this point, after being shown their MRI of the tear, they understand the medical necessity of the procedure to repair the labrum arthroscopically.

SURGICAL TREATMENT:

Arthroscopic Surgery: The most common surgical approach for SLAP lesions.

We make punctures in the skin after sterile preparation in the "beach chair" position. Usually, four punctures (portals) are used to perform the procedure.

Diagnostic arthroscopy is done thoroughly to confirm the diagnosis by direct observation and palpation with a probe.

Debridement and trimming or removing the damaged part of the labrum using a motorized shaver or mechanical biter is done in most cases. Frequently, a large fragment needs removal.

Burring of bone under the labrum is done next to prepare the bed to receive the repaired labrum.

Reattachment is the final step using a suture anchor or two or three.

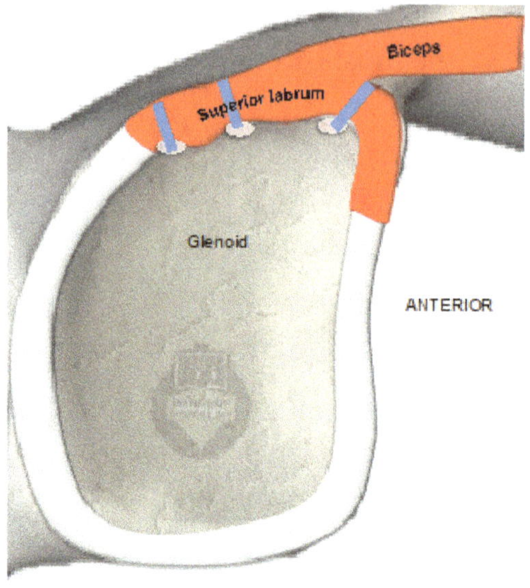

Fig. 5.2.1 Arthroscopic SLAP Repair

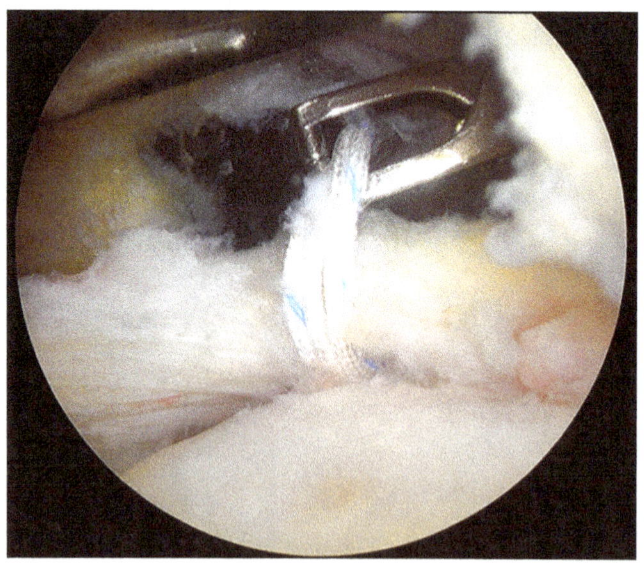

Fig. 5.2.2 SLAP Repair

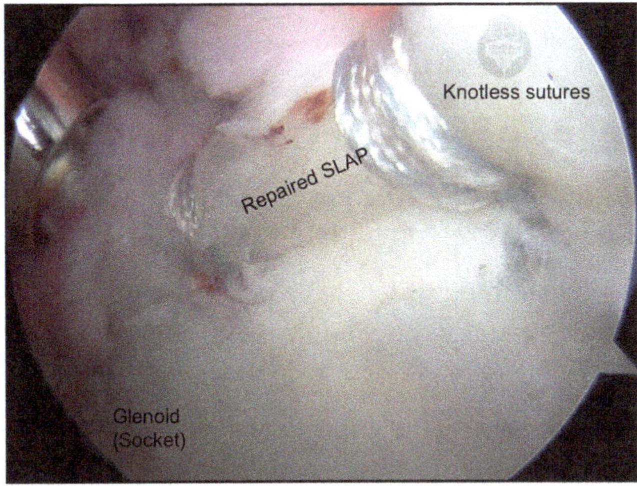

Fig. 5.2.3 SLAP Repair

Labral Repair: Reattaching the torn labrum to the glenoid using anchors and sutures. This part of the procedure is very technical and relies on the use of specific anchors with sutures attached and should be performed by an experienced shoulder arthroscopic surgeon.

Biceps Tenodesis or Tenotomy: If the long head of the biceps tendon is involved, it may be reattached to a different part of the groove of the humeral head (tenodesis). Another option in an older low-use individual is to do a cutting of the tendon (tenotomy).

POST-SURGICAL REHABILITATION:

Immobilization of the shoulder is often done in a sling for several weeks to protect the repair.

Physical Therapy. Gradual progression from passive to active range of motion, followed by strengthening exercises were used in all of my cases. Full recovery takes several months.

A full return to normal activities usually follows the extensive physical therapy program. Especially in athletes who are pitchers or throwing athletes, a gradual and slow specific program is recommended.

CONSIDERATIONS FOR TREATMENT CHOICE:

Age and Activity Level: Younger, active patients, especially athletes, are more likely to undergo surgery.

Severity of Lesion: High-grade lesions or those associated with other shoulder injuries may require surgical intervention.

Failed Conservative Treatment: If non-surgical treatment fails to improve symptoms, surgery may be recommended.

BANKART LESION

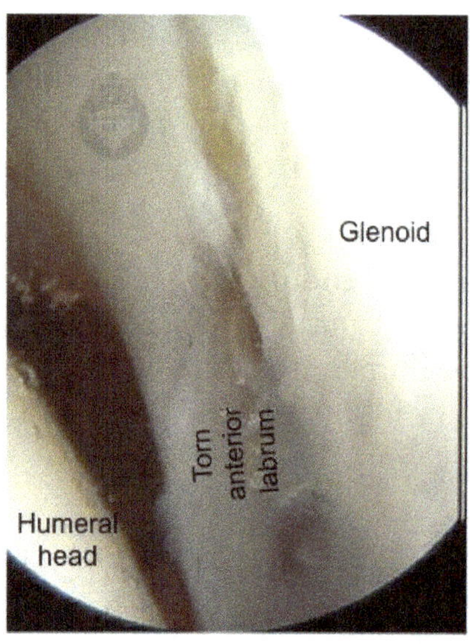

Fig. 5.3.1 Bankart Lesion

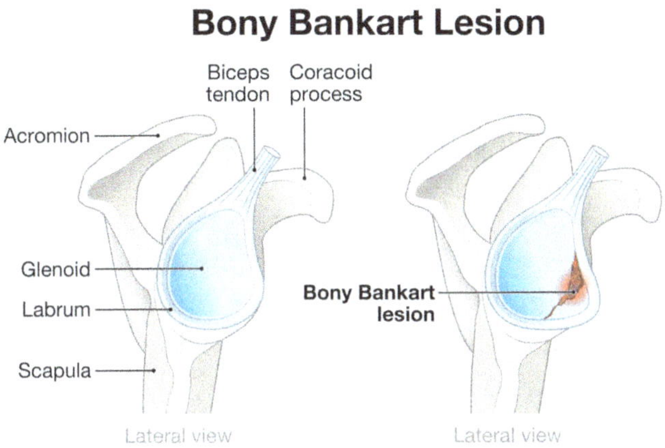

Bony Bankart Lesion

Fig. 5.3.2 Bankart Lesion

A **Bankart lesion** is an injury to the anteroinferior (front-bottom) portion of the glenoid labrum, which is the same ring of cartilage that surrounds the socket of the shoulder joint. This injury often occurs due to anterior shoulder dislocation, where the head of the humerus (upper arm bone) is forced out of the socket, tearing the labrum in the process.

SYMPTOMS AND HISTORY

Patients with this condition often describe a feeling that their shoulder is" going out of place". If it is not the first dislocation, but a subsequent dislocation or subluxation it may happen infrequently or very often. There may be in fact recurrent anterior dislocations if the labrum is very detached and the anterior glenoid bone starts to wear away.

The usual history of this type of patient is one episode where the shoulder actually dislocates and is put back in place. Then at some subsequent event they could be simply relaxing, sleeping, or placing the shoulder in an awkward position. That can cause the shoulder to dislocate. In many cases the shoulder feels as though it's going to go out, but does not completely go out. This is called subluxation.

CLINICAL EXAM

Anterior dislocation. When I examine patients with subluxation or dislocations in the office, moving the shoulder and arm in an external rotation and abducted/extended position causes the patient to tighten up to protect the shoulder. This **Apprehension Test** is an excellent demonstration of the patient protecting the humeral head from going out of the glenoid. The patient has this uneasy feeling that the shoulder joint is going to dislocate. They don't like it.

Another test to determine stability anteriorly in the shoulder is the **Load and Shift Test.** In this test I stabilize the scapula and move the humeral head anteriorly and posteriorly. I can feel the humeral head moving out of the glenoid with this maneuver. The test is said to be positive if there is an excess of translation of the humeral compared to the other side.

Posterior dislocation. It should be noted that there are **posterior dislocations** of the humeral head out of the glenoid but this is much more uncommon than anterior dislocations. I will not discuss posterior dislocations in detail other than stating that there's a tearing of the posterior glenoid and capsule in order for the humeral head to dislocate. The clinical symptoms are pain and tenderness posteriorly and usually these dislocations do not recur in that patient and rarely need surgery

IMAGING STUDIES:

X-rays. Are used primarily to rule out fractures or other bony abnormalities and wearing away of the inferior glenoid rim.

MRI with Arthrogram. This is the gold standard for diagnosing a Bankart lesion. The MRI arthrography involves injecting a contrast dye Gadolinium into the patient's vein, which helps to better visualize the labrum and any associated tears.

CT Scans. These are occasionally used to assess the extent of bony involvement, especially if there is concern about a bony Bankart lesion, where a fragment of the glenoid rim is also broken off anteriorly and inferiorly.

DIAGNOSIS

Now that we have an accurate diagnosis of a **Bankart lesion** which is a tear of the anterior inferior glenoid rim, we can proceed with treatment. In many cases there is some wear of the underlying glenoid bone, and if this is the case and there's a large tear conservative management will not suffice. I do however, recommend to begin with conservative treatment, and proceed to surgical treatment if this fails. Any treatment given needs to be safe, efficient, and effective for the patient to get the best outcome of stability without pain in the shoulder joint.

TREATMENT OF A BANKART LESION

NON-OPERATIVE TREATMENT:

Non-operative management is typically reserved for patients with minimal symptoms or those who are poor surgical risks.This approach includes rest, immobilization, and physical therapy. I often recommend oral anti-inflammatory agents to reduce pain. These are combined with a mixture of corticosteroid, Marcaine, and lidocaine injections. These corticosteroid injections can be given up to three times in a period of approximately three to six months.

Physical Therapy is focused on strengthening the rotator cuff and scapular muscles. These are stabilizers to improve shoulder stability. Range of motion has to be limited to forward flexion and internal rotation and less toward abduction or extension. This is to prevent redislocation or even subluxation during therapy. Use of Theraband in these safe directions is an excellent form of strengthening exercise. Lightweights also should be used for flexion and internal rotation direction. Therapy three times a week is ideal until either maximum stability is achieved. If not then surgery is indicated.

SURGICAL TREATMENT:

Arthroscopic Bankart Repair: The most common treatment for symptomatic Bankart lesions, especially in young, active individuals or athletes. In this procedure, the surgeon uses small incisions to insert instruments into the shoulder joint. The viewing arthroscope is attached to a camera and TV monitor. The torn labrum is reattached to the glenoid rim using special suture anchors.

Open Bankart Repair: In some cases, an open surgery may be performed, which involves a larger incision anteriorly and direct visualization of the labrum for repair. This approach is less common but may be used in complex cases.

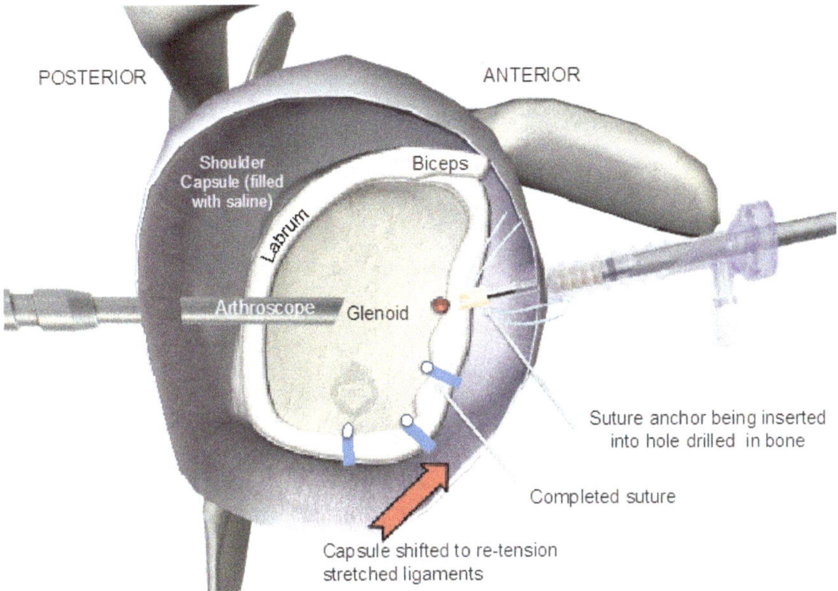

Fig. 5.4.1 Arthroscopic Bankart Repair

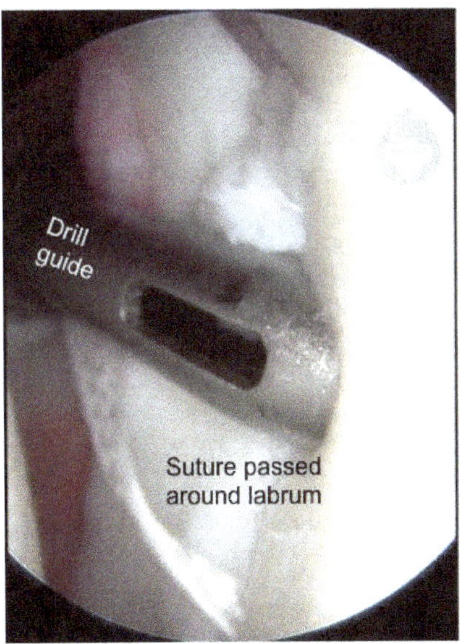

Fig. 5.4.2 Arthroscopic Bankart Repair

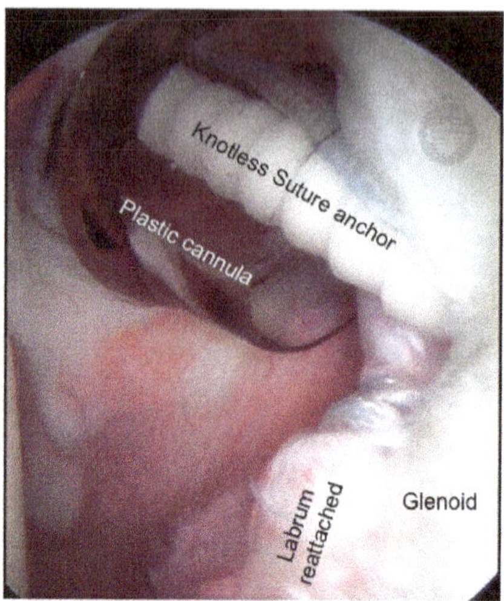

Fig. 5.4.3 Arthroscopic Bankart Repair

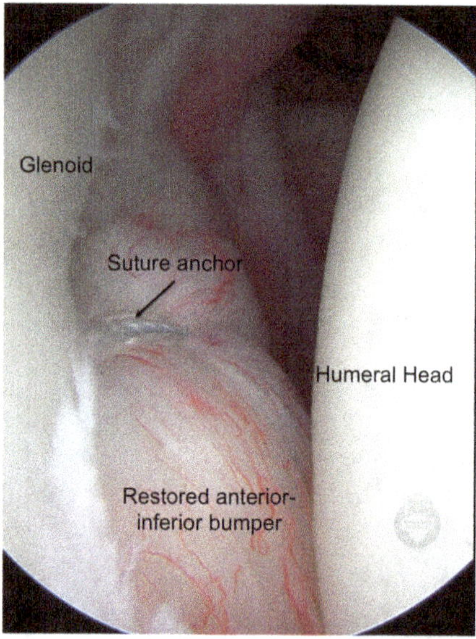

Fig. 5.4.4 Arthroscopic Bankart Repair

POSTOPERATIVE THERAPY:

Immobilization: The shoulder is typically immobilized in a sling for 3-6 weeks postoperatively to allow the labrum to heal. The duration depends on the surgeon's preference and the specifics of the repair.

Early Rehabilitation (0-6 weeks): Focuses on gentle range of motion exercises to prevent stiffness while avoiding excessive stress on the repaired labrum. Passive and assisted range of motion exercises are initiated within a protected range. Extension and external rotation are to be avoided at first. Gradually, directions are introduced.

Intermediate Phase (6-12 weeks): Active range of motion exercises are introduced, and strengthening exercises for the rotator cuff and scapular stabilizers are gradually initiated. The emphasis is on restoring shoulder mobility and stability.

Advanced Strengthening (12-20 weeks): Progressive resistance exercises are incorporated, focusing on regaining full shoulder strength and endurance. Proprioceptive and neuromuscular training is also emphasized.

Return to Sports (5-6 months): Full return to contact sports or overhead activities is usually allowed at 5-6 months post-surgery, assuming the patient has regained full strength, range of motion, and stability.

PROGNOSIS

The prognosis after **Bankart Repair** is generally good, with a high rate of return to pre-injury levels of activity, especially in athletes. However, the risk of recurrence of instability is higher in younger patients, particularly those involved in contact sports.

6 FROZEN SHOULDER AND ADHESIVE CAPSULITIS

Frozen shoulder. Adhesive capsulitis

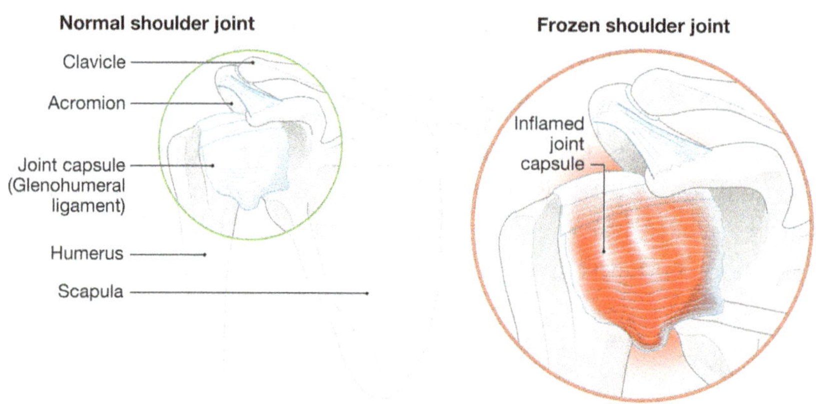

Fig. 6.1 Adhesive Capsulitis

THIS IS A CONDITION CHARACTERIZED BY SEVERE STIFFNESS AND pain in the shoulder joint. It progresses through three stages: **freezing, frozen**, and **thawing** phases. Each stage can last for months and causes progressively worsening pain and loss of motion, followed by gradual recovery. This is much more common in women, in my experience.

CLINICAL SYMPTOMS AND HISTORY

The diagnosis of frozen shoulder is primarily clinical and based on history and physical examination. There is a gradual onset of pain: Often felt deep in the shoulder, typically worse at night and with certain movements.

There is progressive stiffness. There is loss of both active and passive range of motion, particularly external rotation and abduction.

There may be a history of risk factors such as Diabetes, thyroid disorders, or post-surgical immobilization are common risk factors. These

PHYSICAL EXAMINATION

There is a decreased active and passive range of motion: Both the patient and the examiner are unable to move the shoulder beyond a certain **capsular pattern restriction**: Most notably, loss of external rotation occurs.

IMAGING STUDIES

X-rays are generally normal but may be used to rule out other causes (e.g., arthritis).

MRI or Ultrasound are not typically required but can show thickening of the shoulder joint capsule or rule out other pathologies (e.g., rotator cuff tears).

DIAGNOSIS

With the diagnosis of **adhesive capsulitis** being made, we can proceed with treatment. The problem of dense scar tissue in the capsule needs to be addressed primarily. Safe, efficient treatment with a good outcome is the goal. Unfortunately, in some cases the goal of full range of painless movement is not achieved.

TREATMENT

The goal of treatment is to **reduce pain** and **restore range of motion**. Treatment varies by stage and severity:

NON-SURGICAL TREATMENT

Medication is used to reduce pain and inflammation. There usually is pain once therapy starts. The use of non steroid anti-inflammatory drugs is typical of treatment. Sleeping medication, I believe, is also helpful due to pain worsening at night. Corticosteroids by injection combined with lidocaine and Marcaine are also very helpful to reduce pain and inflammation. Injections are placed in the subacromial space. These injections can be done up to three times in a three to six month.

Physical Therapy. The mainstay of treatment is to restore motion. Gentle, progressive stretching exercises tailored to the stage of the condition. A very important component in gaining range of motion is patient tolerance. We all have a threshold for pain. During therapy even the gentlest therapist will cause pain. Pain meds and injections will help.

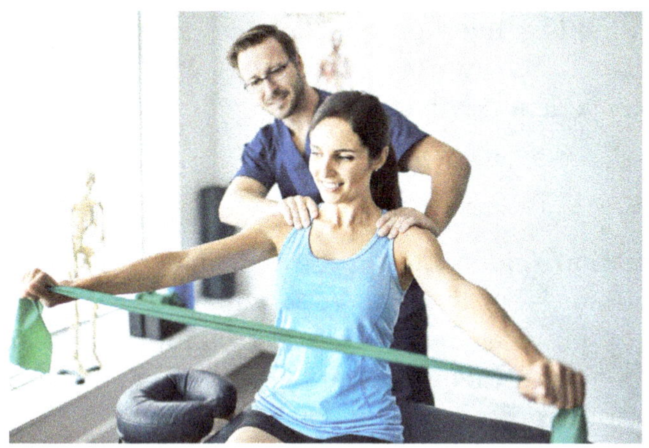

Fig. 6.2 Theraband Stretching and Strengthening

Non-Steroidal Anti-Inflammatory Drugs (NSAIDs). To reduce pain and inflammation. these can easily be obtained over the counter and there are many different choices depending on the patient's response to substances such as ibuprofen, naproxen, or others. Acetaminophen can be used to alleviate pain.

Corticosteroid Injections. Intra-articular corticosteroid injections may be effective in the early, painful phases to reduce inflammation and speed recovery. These injections are also helpful during the phase of physical therapy because the movement by the therapist can cause a great deal of inflammation. As noted earlier these can be given over a three to six month period.

Warm Swimming Therapy. Ideally, in my experience, the use of a warm swimming pool on a daily basis is of great benefit. Initially, using a breaststrok, sidestrokel, followed by the butterfly stroke ultimately worked very well for the majority of my patients with this problem. The water is warm and gentle; it numbs up the pain, allowing the patient to do their workout easier. This has been the best tool in all of my cases where the shoulder range of motion has to be re-achieved.

Hydrodilatation. Injection of saline and steroids to stretch the joint capsule and improve mobility is used in some cases. I have no experience with this technique personally.

SURGICAL TREATMENT

Manipulation under anesthesia is usually necessary because the scar tissue is so strong and dense that it cannot be stretched or torn by physical therapy alone. It is too painful when the patient is awake. Light general anesthesia is used to first lyse (cut) the adhesions and gain maximum range of motion. In most cases arthroscopic surgery is necessary to clean out and cauterize the scar tissue that was just torn or cut. This is done at the same time under the same general anesthetic.

Manipulation under Anesthesia (MUA): In all cases I have treated I have forcibly but safely and smoothly moved the shoulder while the patient is under general anesthesia to break up adhesions and improve range of motion. I could feel the crackeling of the scar tissue as I felt the giving way of the tightness of the shoulder. I would push posteriorly first in a rotational fashion as illustrated in **Fig.6**. Afterward I would then move the shoulder in a lateral position getting, if possible, the full range of motion.

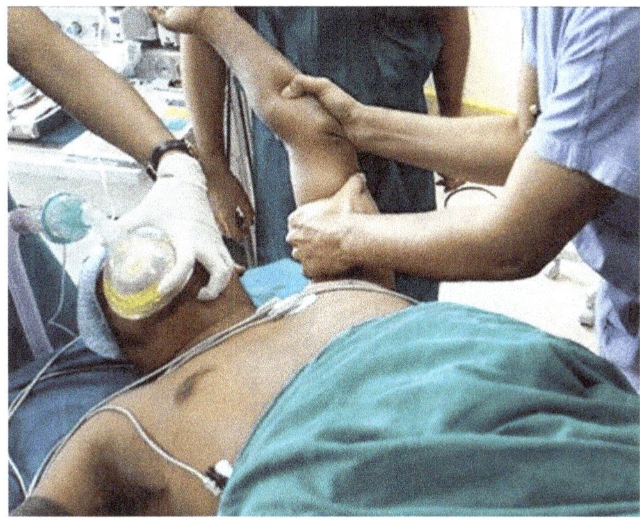

Fig. 6.3 Manipulation Under Anesthesia of Frozen a
Frozen Shoulder

Arthroscopic Capsular Release: Minimally invasive surgery where the tight, thickened capsule is cut to release the joint and allow better motion. After the manipulation or anesthesia breaks up the scar tissue with audible and palpable crepitus, the shoulder has three punctures made in it, and an arthroscope is introduced to view the inside, and other punctures are used for cutting and shaving instruments.

Under direct vision, the scar tissue that broke up is then removed with the cutting-sucking instrument called the shaver, and the Electrocautery is used to stop any bleeders. The cautery prevents the recurrence of scar tissue forming.

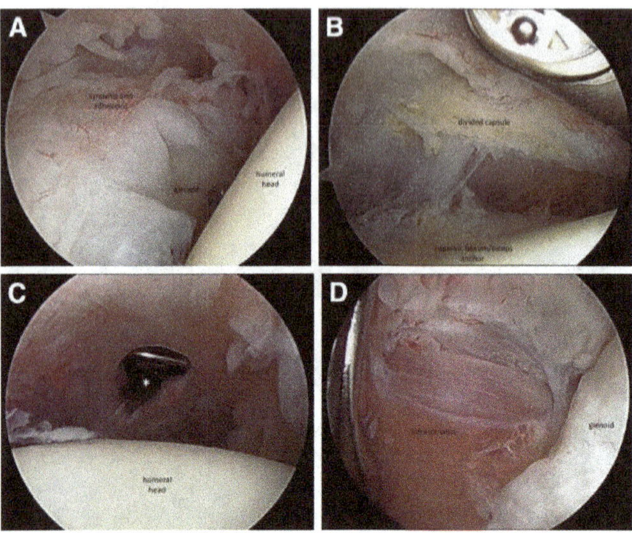

Fig. 6.4 Arthroscopic Lysis of Adhesions

Once completed, each of the punctures is closed with one suture after irrigating the joint with the antibiotic solution to prevent infection. An injection of hydrocortisone derivative, lidocaine, and Marcaine is put in the shoulder for post-op pain relief. The steroid helps reduce the inflammation and the reformation of scar tissue. It should be noted that the shoulder needs to be moved early after surgery so it does not tighten up and scar down again. If available, a CPM machine is utilized. This machine is set up at the home and moves the shoulder passively 24/7. This CPM machine moves the shoulder gently and continuously and helps achieve a more rapid range of motion.

PROGNOSIS

Frozen shoulder with appropriate treatment typically resolves over time, but can take **12–24 months**. Most patients regain functional range of motion, although complete recovery of full motion may not always occur. Early intervention and aggressive physical therapy can help reduce long-term stiffness. Most moderate to severe cases require Manipulation Under Anesthesia followed by Arthroscopic cleanout of adhesions.

7 COMMON CHALLENGES AND COMPLICATIONS OF ARTHROSCOPIC

ROTATOR CUFF REPAIR

Some of the most common include:

1. Retear or Failure of the Repair

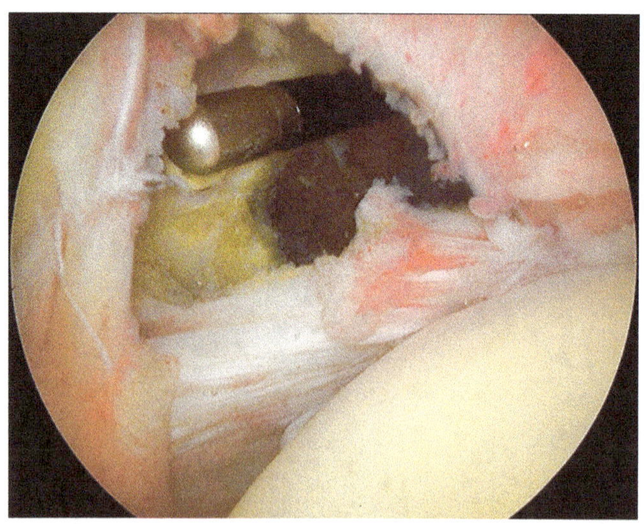

Fig.7.1 Muscle Tendon Pullout

High Retear Rates: In spite of successful surgery done technically and despite advancements in techniques and materials, rotator cuff repairs have a relatively high retear rate, especially in larger or massive tears. This is often due to poor tissue quality, tendon degeneration, or patient non-compliance during rehabilitation.

Biomechanical Challenges: The rotator cuff's complex anatomy and high mechanical stress make repairs challenging. Achieving proper tendon-to-bone healing can be difficult, especially when tendon quality is poor.

STIFFNESS AND LOSS OF RANGE OF MOTION

Postoperative stiffness is a common issue, sometimes due to adhesions or poor rehabilitation. If the shoulder isn't mobilized appropriately after surgery, stiffness can develop, leading to restricted motion.

Patients who overprotect the shoulder during early recovery may experience more stiffness, while those who are too aggressive may cause re-tearing.

INFECTION

Infection is a risk with any surgery, although the rate for rotator cuff repair is relatively low. When it does occur, it can lead to poor healing, chronic pain, and the need for additional surgery.

CHRONIC PAIN

Even with successful tendon healing, some patients may experience persistent pain. This could be due to residual inflammation, irritation of surrounding structures, or a failure of complete tendon integration.

TENDON RETRACTION AND MUSCLE ATROPHY

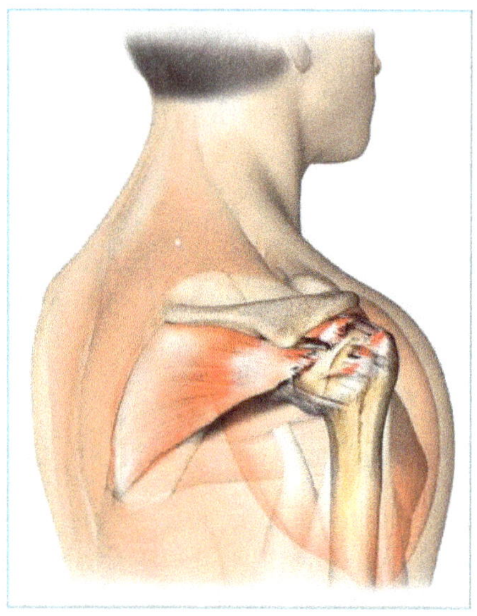

Fig. 7.2 Severe Muscle Retraction

Chronic rotator cuff tears often result in tendon retraction and muscle atrophy, which can complicate surgical repair. Reattaching a retracted tendon can be difficult, and the muscle may not regain full strength postoperatively.

NERVE DAMAGE

Although rare, there is a risk of nerve injury during the surgery. This could lead to weakness or loss of sensation in the arm or shoulder.

FAILURE OF GRAFT OR AUGMENTATION

In cases where tissue grafts or synthetic materials are used to augment the repair, these materials may fail to integrate properly or provide the intended support.

ADHESIVE CAPSULITIS (FROZEN SHOULDER)

This condition, marked by stiffness and pain, can develop either before or after surgery. It may require additional physical therapy or even surgery to correct it.

COMPLICATIONS RELATED TO HARDWARE

When anchors, screws, or other hardware are used to reattach the tendon to bone, there is a risk of mechanical failure, loosening, or migration of the hardware, which may necessitate revision surgery.

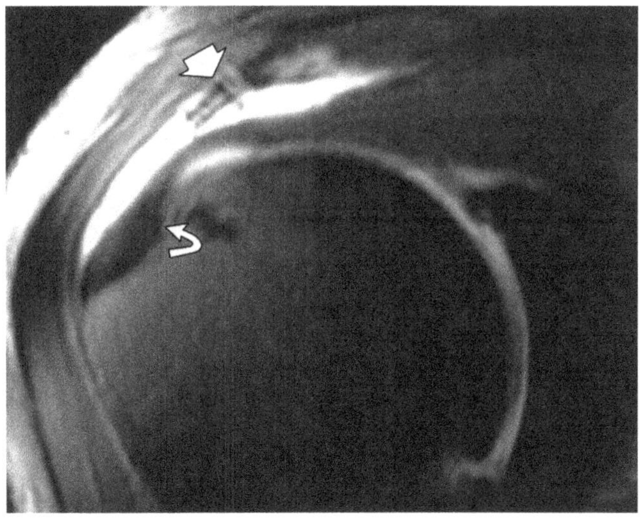

Fig. 7.3 Loosened Hardware a Screw Anchor

Minimizing these risks requires careful surgical technique, proper patient selection, and a well-structured rehabilitation program.

Biceps Long Head (LH) Rupture. Occasionally, the biceps tendon LH is so worn out and inflamed that it is definitely contributing to the pain in the shoulder. It is so thin and worn that during a rotator cuff repair, it can rupture during surgery. Also just due to the attenuation of the tendon itself it can rupture. This has to be dealt with by tenodesis usually, or in some cases it can be just a tenotomy or cutting the tendon. My preference is tenodesis.

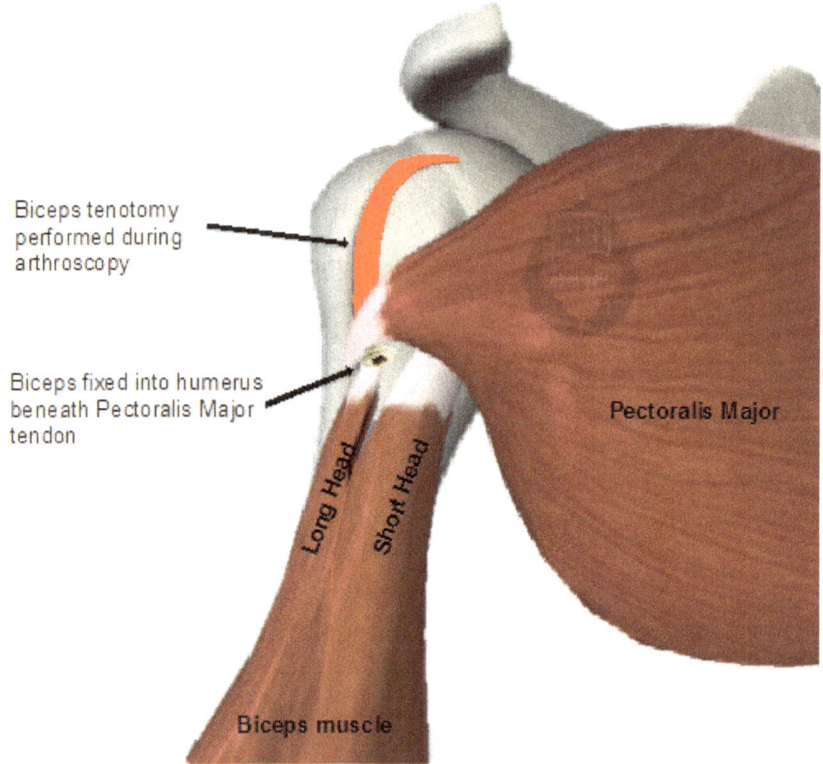

Fig. 7.4 Biceps Tendonitis/ Rupture

Persistent Pain. Some patients may experience ongoing pain despite a technically successful surgery, which can be due to various factors like incomplete repair, nerve irritation, or concomitant shoulder pathology such as arthritis. Thorough preoperative evaluation addressing all potential sources of pain during surgery and comprehensive postoperative management is necessary for treatment.

Failure to return to pre-injury activity levels. Some patients may not regain the full strength or functionality required for their previous level of sports or occupational activities. Realistic goal-setting, patient education, and a well-structured, gradual return to activity physical therapy program are absolutely necessary to avoid this complication.

PHYSICAL THERAPY PROGRAM TO OPTIMIZE ROTATOR CUFF SURGERY

This is an outline of a physical therapy program for a pitcher or quarterback who needs to return to a throwing sport or a worker with a job that requires a high level of performance of the shoulders.

PHASE 1: ACUTE PHASE (0-2 WEEKS POST-INJURY)

Goals: Control inflammation, manage pain, maintain range of motion (ROM), and begin light strengthening.

- **Rest and Protection:** Avoid throwing or overhead activities.
- **Ice and Anti-inflammatory Techniques:** Apply ice for 15-20 minutes every 2-3 hours.
- **ROM Exercises:**
  - Pendulum exercises
  - Passive and active-assisted shoulder ROM (flexion, abduction, external rotation)
- **Isometric Strengthening:**
  - Shoulder isometrics (flexion, extension, abduction, internal/external rotation)
  - Scapular stabilization exercises (scapular squeezes)
- **Core Activation:** Light core exercises such as pelvic tilts and planks.

PHASE 2: INTERMEDIATE PHASE (3-6 WEEKS POST-INJURY)

Goals: Restore full ROM, improve strength, and begin neuromuscular control.

- **Advanced ROM Exercises:**
  - Full active shoulder ROM in all planes
  - Gentle stretching for internal and external rotation
- **Strengthening:**
  - Resistance band exercises (rows, external/internal rotation)
  - Scapular stabilization (Y, T, W exercises)
  - Rotator cuff strengthening
- **Core and Lower Body Strengthening:**
  - Progressive core exercises (Russian twists, medicine ball throws)
  - Lower body strengthening (lunges, squats)
- **Neuromuscular Control:**
  - Rhythmic stabilization exercises
  - PNF patterns with a focus on proprioception

PHASE 3: ADVANCED STRENGTHENING AND NEUROMUSCULAR TRAINING (7-10 WEEKS POST-INJURY)

Goals: Achieve full strength and endurance, enhance dynamic stability, and begin sport-specific drills.

- **Dynamic Strengthening:**
  - Weight training focused on shoulder, scapula, and core (overhead presses, push-ups)
  - Plyometric exercises (medicine ball slams, push-ups with claps)
- **Dynamic Neuromuscular Control:**
  - Advanced PNF patterns with resistance

- ○ Balance and stability exercises (single-leg balance, Bosu ball drills)
- **Functional Drills:**
  - ○ Throwing progression with light implements
  - ○ Sport-specific movements without full load

PHASE 4: RETURN TO SPORT (11+ WEEKS POST-INJURY) OR VIGOROUS JOB

Goals: Gradual return to full throwing activity, enhance performance, and prevent reinjury.

- **Throwing Program:**
  - ○ Begin with short, controlled throws
  - ○ Gradually increase distance, intensity, and frequency
  - ○ Monitor for any signs of pain or fatigue
- **Sport-Specific Conditioning:**
  - ○ Agility drills, sprints, and quick direction changes
  - ○ Full-body conditioning focusing on sport-specific demands
- **Plyometric and Power Training:**
  - ○ High-intensity plyometrics (box jumps, rotational throws)
  - ○ Powerlifting techniques under supervision
- **Mental Conditioning:**
  - ○ Visualization techniques
  - ○ Gradual reintegration into team practice
- **Final Return:**
  - ○ Participate in non-contact drills, progressing to full contact or high-intensity practices.
  - ○ Continue monitoring shoulder mechanics to ensure proper form and avoid overuse.

MAINTENANCE PROGRAM

- **Strengthening and Flexibility:** Continue shoulder and core exercises 2-3 times per week.
- **Injury Prevention:** Regular mobility work, scapular stability, and neuromuscular control exercises.
- **Recovery Strategies:** Adequate rest, hydration, and nutrition, along with consistent use of recovery modalities (ice, massage, etc.).

It should be said that in my experience of over four decades of rotator cuff surgery, this is a challenge for any surgeon because each case is unique. The patient's tissues are unique, the stresses after the repair are unique, and they are all, in my experience, a challenge. An optimal physical therapy program, good nutrition and cooperation between the surgeon and the patient are absolutely required to achieve an excellent result and avoid complications.

8 ACROMIO-CLAVICULAR (AC) SEPARATIONS AND ARTHRITIS

DESCRIPTION OF INJURY

Injury to the AC joint, where the Clavicle (collarbone) meets the Acromion (part of the Scapula) at the lateral point of the shoulder.

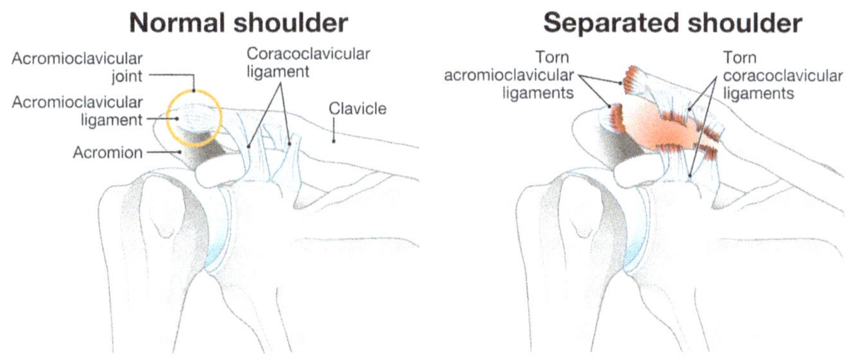

Fig. 8.1 Acromioclavicular Separation

The AC joint connecting the clavicle to the Acromion portion of the Scapula provides a bony framework for the attachment of muscles. These bones also provide the protection for the glenohumeral portion of the shoulder joint as well as vessels and nerves.

Various forces, such as a direct fall on the point of the shoulder or a force from the back or the front of the clavicle to the acromion, can tear two sets of ligaments. One set of ligaments is the **Acromioclavicular Ligament**. The other set is the **Coracoclavicular Ligament.** Depending on which ligaments are torn, these injuries have been classified as noted below.

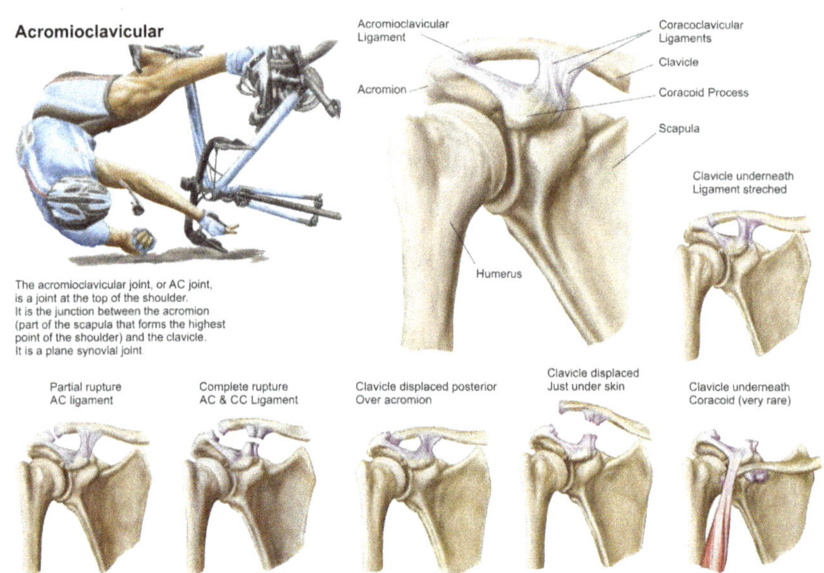

Fig. 8.1.1 A-C Classification and Mechanism of Injury

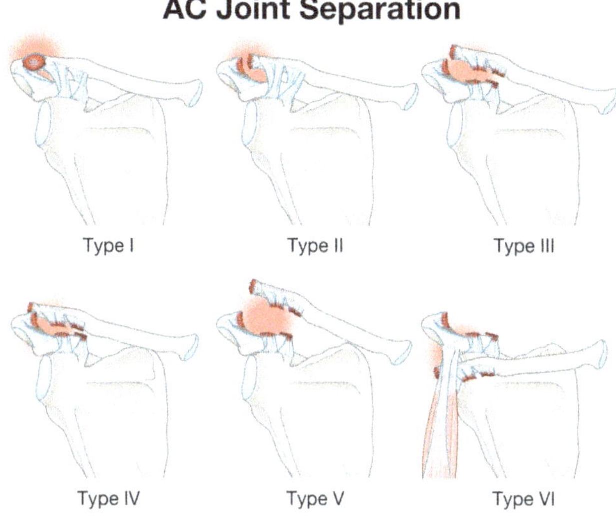

Fig. 8.1.2 A-C Separation Classification Anatomy

CLASSIFICATION:

1. **Type I:** Sprain of the A-C ligament without displacement.
2. **Type II:** Tear of the A-C ligament, partial displacement.
3. **Type III:** Complete tear of A-C and coracoclavicular (CC) ligaments, full displacement.
4. **Type IV:** Complete tear with posterior displacement of the clavicle.
5. **Type V:** Severe displacement with significant disruption of the deltotrapezial fascia.
6. **Type VI:** Inferior displacement of the clavicle (very rare).

MECHANISM OF INJURY:

Direct blow to the shoulder. In sports such as football, soccer, hockey, skiing, snowboarding, gymnastics, bicycling, and basketball. Injury can happen in any activity that one can think of where there is a forceful exposure of the shoulder joint. These forces would disrupt the ligaments that connect the clavicle to the acromion and the coracoid process

Fall onto the shoulder or outstretched hand. The most common mechanism of injury is a fall onto the point of the shoulder, such as to the side or to the front. Or a fall with the handout stretched, putting all the forces up into the shoulder joint, which can cause an AC separation.

SYMPTOMS AND HISTORY

There is a **visible bump or deformity at the AC joint** immediately after the fall or trauma. There is an obvious painful swelling or bump at the top of the shoulder. There is also immediate pain at the top of the shoulder, and this can occur sometimes with a delay of 10 to 15 minutes as swelling and bleeding develop.

Swelling and bruising. This initial swelling is sometimes associated with immediate bleeding and, therefore, discoloration of the skin, but deep bruising doesn't occur until hours later as the bleeding, which is deep, comes gradually to the surface of the skin. This bruising also drifts down into the arm and forearm due to gravity.

Limited shoulder movement. In the beginning, the shoulder does not move normally. It can be either completely frozen in pain, or it may move a little, but it is extremely painful when movement does occur. The pain can usually be located in the A-C joint on the top of the shoulder, but it can also radiate either down into the hand or up into the neck.

Physical examination. The first step in diagnosis is the physical examination. The obvious presence of a bump, bruising, or swelling, as noted earlier, is the initial physical observation associated with the patient's complaint of pain and limited motion. Upon palpation of the shoulder, occasionally, one can even feel the separation of the clavicle from the acromion with a space of approximately 1 centimeter at times. Generally, it's just swollen and bruised and very tender to touch. Making an attempt to range the motion by moving the arm at all causes exquisite pain and complaints by the patient.

X-rays (stress views may be needed). The next step, especially in the first shoulder injuries with dislocation or subluxation of the A-C joint, is X-rays. X-rays can reveal the displacement of the clavicle from the acromion but also fractures that may not be appreciated from a simple examination.

Occasionally, **stress X-rays** are required. While the patient is having the X-ray taken in an upright position (either standing or sitting), he is holding a 5 LB sandbag. This X-ray technique distracts acromion from the clavicle. This test is done when this separation is suspected but does not appear obvious on plane X-ray.

MRI. Also, in some cases, especially when a rotator cuff tear is suspected and needs to be ruled out along with the A-C separation, MRIs are indicated. The MRI demonstrates the torn ligaments, both the Acromioclavicular Ligament on top and the deep Coracoclavicular Ligament. With these studies, a complete picture of the shoulder injury is obtained.

DIAGNOSIS

Once the diagnosis of **Acromioclavicular Separation** is made treatment can be planned. Based on the degree of injury and classification I-VI a choice from conservative to surgical treatment plan is undertaken.

NON-OPERATIVE TREATMENT:

Type I and II: Conservative management (rest, ice, NSAIDs, physical therapy). For the treatment of type I and type II AC joint injuries where there is tearing of the Acromioclavicular Ligament, both minimally sprained and somewhat stretched, conservative treatment is highly recommended.

The patient's arm is put into a sling to unweight the arm from pulling down on the shoulder. Also, a figure-of-eight brace should be applied to pull the clavicle down toward the acromion. Both of these are available commercially or through an orthopedic surgeon or a physical therapist. These braces or slings should be worn for approximately four to six weeks even though the A-C joint feels better probably after two or three weeks. This allows healing time for the ligaments to maintain strength, length, and tightness.

Type III: It is controversial and can be treated conservatively or surgically. In type III, there is a tearing not only of the Acromioclavicular Ligament but, more importantly, the Coracoclavicular Ligament. When both of these ligaments are torn, there can be 2 or 3mm displacement all the way up to 2 cm of displacement of the clavicle up from the acromion.

Depending on the sport the need for a complete reconnection of the clavicle to the acromion, surgery may be indicated. In some sports, such as football, where the quarterback has to use his arm to throw during the season, if the injury occurs early, the A-C joint is not fixed until the end of the season. At the end of the season the more major operation can be performed at that time.

The repair of the A-C joint is done with pins or a plate occasionally. A graft is used to improve both the function and the cosmesis of the shoulder joint. If a joint is left unoperated and unstable, weakness, chronic pain, and sometimes hand and arm numbness can develop.

SURGICAL TREATMENT

The decision to operate on a A-C separation III is a critical one and needs to be made between the surgeon and the patient as it applies to the sports and work function needed.

Type IV, V, VI: Surgical intervention is always required. Treatment for type IV V or VI AC joint separations is surgical, but once again, if the circumstances, for example, a professional athlete who is a quarterback, occurs early in the season, that procedure will be delayed until a long recovery is allowed for the major surgical procedure required.

SURGERIES FOR A-C SEPARATION OF THE SHOULDER

Acromioclavicular (A-C) joint separation, often caused by trauma or injury, is treated based on the severity of the separation. The surgeries for A-C joint separation range from minimally invasive techniques to more complex procedures. Here are the main types of joint injury.

The surgical management of type III, type IV, type V, and type VI A-C separations, including indications, techniques, and postoperative considerations, is discussed now.

Type III is controversial since there is not a great deal of separation in most cases. There is a belief among many orthopedic surgeons that if a type III separation is not repaired, then future post-traumatic arthritis of the A-C joint will develop. Indications also include the need for high-demand use of the shoulder, such as in many athletes and laborers. In patients who are concerned with the cosmetic appearance of their shoulder from the bump in an unrepaired A-C separation, surgery is also indicated.

Type IV through type VI is generally recommended due to

significant displacement and dysfunction, including neurological deficit that occurs.

SURGICAL TECHNIQUES USED TO REPAIR THE A-C SEPARATIONS III-VI

1. Open Reduction and Internal Fixation (ORIF)

Procedure: Involves making a 5-6 cm incision over the A-C joint to directly visualize and repair the ligaments. Various methods are available to bring the clavicle down to the acromion with fixation.

A-C SURGICAL SHOULDER REPAIRS

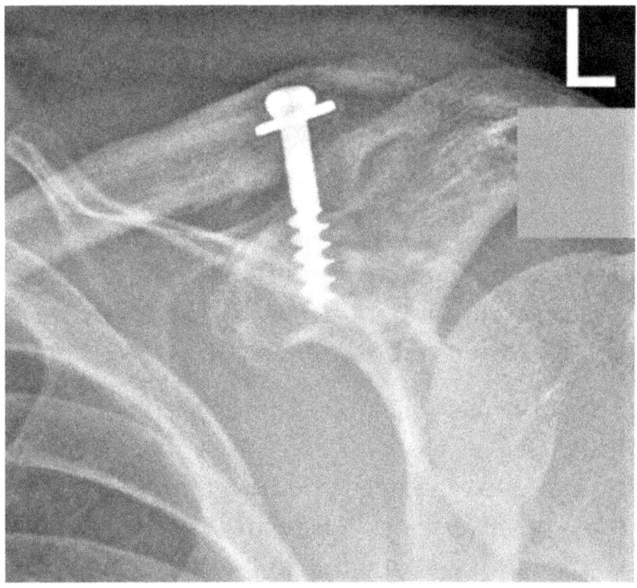

Fig. 8.2.1 Bosworth Screw

A special **Bosworth Screw** is utilized and this is drilled through the clavicle and into the coracoid process and this is done usually is an open procedure or through a minimal incision.

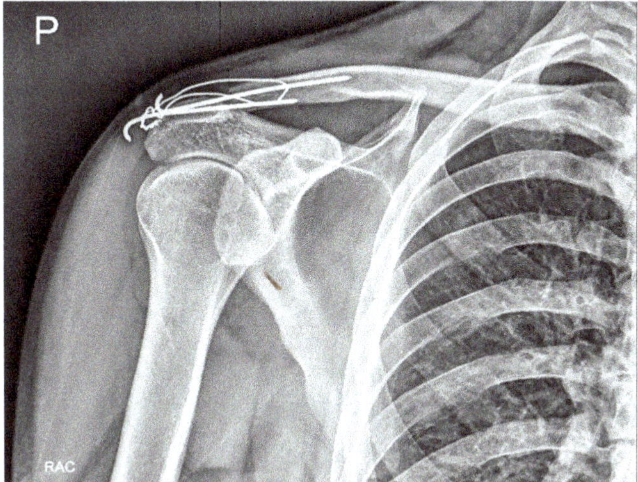

Fig. 8.2.2 Intramedullary Rod

Pins or small rods are placed in the acromion and into the clavicle to stabilize the joint; it can be supplemented by wires as well.

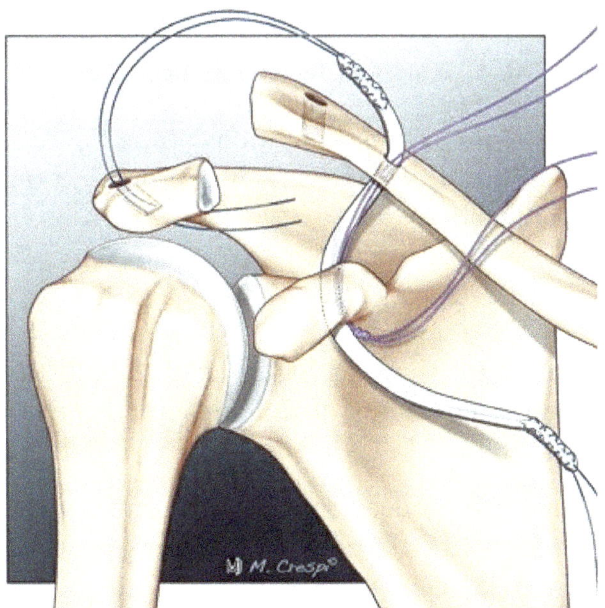

Fig. 8.2.3 Fascial Loop Around Coracoid and Clavicle

ALLOGRAFT OR AUTOGRAFT IN RECONSTRUCTIONS OPEN PROCEDURE

Procedure: Uses graft tissue from the patient (autograft) or a donor (allograft) to reconstruct the damaged ligaments.

The **Fascial Graft** is woven around the Clavicle and under the Coracoid process and this will bring down the Clavicle into its more anatomical position. This graft stays permanently.

Benefits: This graft provides a strong, durable repair. The patient should have no limitations in throwing activities or very physical use of the shoulder at work.

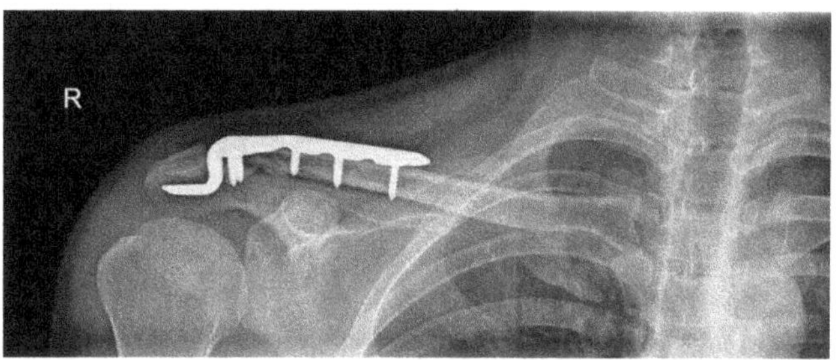

Fig. 8.2.4 Hook Plate Fixation

Indications: More severe separations (Type IV, V, or VI) where there's significant displacement. Some examples are demonstrated below:

HOOKPLATE OPEN

A **Hookplate** with short screws is used to hold the clavicle in place while the ligaments heal. Plates and screws are usually removed.

A **Hookplate** can be used with several screws attached to the clavicle and the hook goes under the acromion and this stabilizes the clavicle to the acromion and this is an extreme technique that is infrequently used in my experience. The plate can be removed at some point in the future.

The advantage of this method is that it provides immediate stability. There still however is a recovery and therapy period.

WEAVER-DUNN PROCEDURE OPEN PREOCEDURE

Procedure: This involves transferring the coracoacromial ligament to the distal end of the clavicle to stabilize the AC joint.

Utilizes the body's natural tissues for repair.Often used for chronic cases or where other procedures have failed

The indications for using this method are severe or complex cases where original ligaments are significantly damaged.

ARTHROSCOPIC SURGERY

Arthroscopy is a minimally invasive surgery involving making small incisions and using an arthroscope to visualize and repair the joint.

The benefits are use of less tissue damage, shorter recovery time, and minimal scarring.

Generally used for less severe separations (Type II or III).

POST-SURGICAL CONSIDERATIONS FOR ALL A-C SURGERIES.

Rehabilitation and **Physical therapy** are essential to restore function and strength.

Recovery Time varies depending on the procedure and the severity of the injury, ranging from a few weeks to several months.

Complications: There is a potential for infection, hardware issues, or incomplete healing.

The choice of surgery depends on factors such as the severity of the injury, patient activity level, and overall health. Consulting with an orthopedic surgeon will help determine the best approach for each individual case.

ACROMIOCLAVICULAR ARTHRITIS

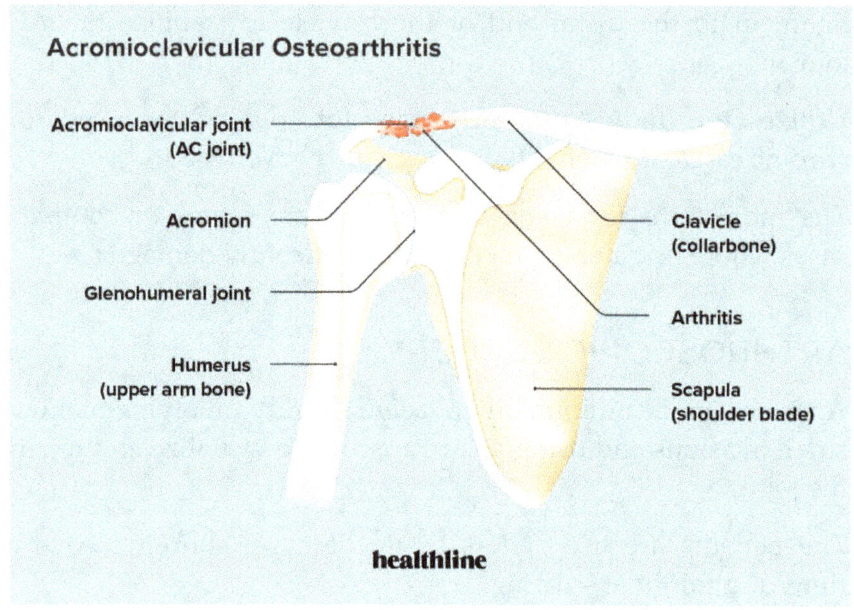

Fig. 8.3 A-C Arthritis

Acromioclavicular (A-C) joint arthritis is a common condition, particularly in middle-aged and older adults or in younger individuals with a history of shoulder trauma or heavy overhead activity. The A-C joint, located at the top of the shoulder where the clavicle (collarbone) meets the acromion (part of the scapula), is prone to wear and tear due to its role in shoulder movement and load-bearing.

CAUSES

Degenerative Arthritis (Osteoarthritis): This is the most common cause of A-C joint arthritis, resulting from the gradual wear and tear of the joint cartilage over time.

Post-Traumatic Arthritis: This can develop after an injury to the shoulder, such as an A-C joint separation or fracture of the distal clavicle.

Inflammatory Arthritis: Conditions like Rheumatoid Arthritis can also affect the A-C joint, although this is less common.

SYMPTOMS

Pain: Typically localized to the top of the shoulder, particularly when reaching across the body, lifting objects overhead, or lying on the affected side.

Swelling and Tenderness: The A-C joint may become tender to the touch and swelling may be present. Frequently, a large obvious bump develops over time.

Reduced Range of Motion: Particularly with movements that involve lifting the arm across the body or overhead progressively the shoulder gradually starts hurting more with movements.Popping is associated with this.

Crepitus: Crepitus the medical term for grating or grinding sensation. This may be felt in the joint during movement. Noise is produced, the grinding and popping can be heard very loudly at times.This is accompanied by pain that ranges from 3/10 to 10/10.

Clinical Examination: A physical exam can reveal tenderness over the A-C joint, pain with specific movements (like the cross-body adduction test), and possible swelling. The obvious bump is classic. Limited motion is also noted due to pain specifically in the A-C joint area.

IMAGING

X-rays can show narrowing of the joint space, osteophytes (bone spurs), and subchondral sclerosis (increased bone density under the cartilage) at the end of the clavicle.

MRI or Ultrasound may be used to assess the joint and surrounding soft tissues in more detail, especially if other shoulder pathologies are suspected such as Impingement and rotator cuff pathology.

DIAGNOSIS

A-C Joint Arthritis is extremely common especially in men who are very physical in their work or in their athletics. Activities such as weight lifting, physical fitness exercises such as push-ups and upper extremity weight lifting causes unusually high stresses on the A-C joint. Throwing sports and racquet sports also contribute a great deal of injury to the A-C joint overtime.

Prior first or second degree or even third degree A-C joint separations with or without surgery can also lead to A-C joint arthritis. There are diseases such as Osteoarthritis or Rheumatoid Arthritis that can cause this condition. Rheumatoid Arthritis occurs somewhat more often in females.

TREATMENT OPTIONS

Primarily because of pain in this arthritic A-C joint patient seeks help. In my experience the most conservative approach is usually beneficial for a period of time, but ultimately in moderate to severe cases of A-C joint arthritis surgery has to be done.

Conservative Management: Reducing activities that exacerbate symptoms, especially overhead or cross-body movements is strongly recommended.

Physical Therapy: Strengthening the muscles around the shoulder and improving shoulder mechanics can help reduce pain and limitation of motion in the A-C joint.

Nonsteroidal Anti-Inflammatory Drugs (NSAIDs): These taken orally can help manage pain and inflammation. Examples of these over the counter medications are naproxen, ibuprofen, and others.

Corticosteroid Injections: An injection into the A-C joint can provide temporary relief from pain and inflammation for weeks to months in my experience. These injections should be used also for both diagnosis and treatment.

SURGICAL TREATMENT

Distal Clavicle Resection (Mumford Procedure): If conservative measures fail, this open procedure involves a 4 cm incision over the A-C joint. Using an osteotome (chisel) a small portion of the distal clavicle is removed, usually 2 cm, to eliminate the painful bone-on-bone contact between the distal clavicle and the acromion of the joint.

It can be done through open surgery as described or arthroscopically. My preference for the last 40 years has been arthroscopic.

Arthroscopic A-C Joint Debridement (Mumford Procedure) This involves cleaning out the joint space, removing loose fragments, and smoothing rough cartilage surfaces. This procedure primarily depends on the use of a bur and irrigation to clear out the bony fragments that are created with the bur. Direct vision is excellent in this procedure. Resection of 2 cm of clavicle should be achieved in every case. If done, this is curative.

PROGNOSIS

With appropriate treatment, many individuals experience complete relief from symptoms. However, ongoing management may be required, especially if underlying degenerative changes are present in other areas of the joint, such as the glenohumeral portion. In cases where surgery is necessary, the outcomes are generally favorable, with a high percentage of patients returning to their previous levels of activity.

Occasionally over many years the distal clavicle regrows bone and the A-C joint is painful again. If very bothersome with pain additional surgery would probably be needed and recommended.

SURGICAL PROCEDURE OUTLINES

The Mumford procedure, also known as distal clavicle resection or distal clavicle excision, is a surgical technique used to treat conditions like A-C joint arthritis, chronic A-C joint pain, or post-traumatic arthritis. The goal is to remove the distal (lateral) 2 cm of the clavicle to eliminate pain caused by bone-on-bone contact with the acromion. This can be done through either an open or arthroscopic approach.

OPEN MUMFORD PROCEDURE (ORIGINAL)

Preoperative Preparation

Anesthesia: General anesthesia or regional anesthesia (such as an interscalene block) is typically used.

Positioning: The patient is placed in a **beach-chair** or semi-recumbent position. The affected arm is draped freely to allow for movement during the procedure.

Surgical Steps Open Procedure

Incision: A small, 3-5 cm incision is made over the A-C joint. This incision is typically horizontal and directly over the joint, allowing easy access to the distal clavicle.

Exposure: The deltotrapezial fascia is incised and retracted, exposing the distal end of the clavicle and the AC joint. Care is taken to preserve the integrity of the fascia for later repair.

Soft tissues around the joint, including the joint capsule, are dissected, cauterized, and retracted to fully expose the distal clavicle.

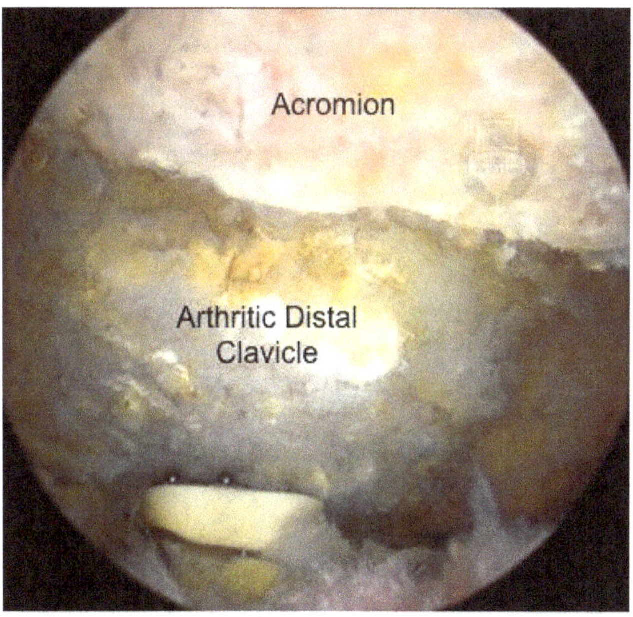

Fig. 8.4.1 Mumford Procedure

Resection of Distal Clavicle: A saw or osteotome is used to remove the distal 2 cm of the clavicle. The amount resected can vary depending on the surgeon's preference and the extent of the pathology, however total contact with the acromion must be eliminated.

The cut end of the clavicle is smoothed to prevent any sharp edges that could irritate surrounding tissues.

Hemostasis: Bleeding is controlled using electrocautery or other hemostatic agents.

Closure: The deltotrapezial fascia is meticulously repaired to ensure stability.

Subcutaneous tissues and skin are closed in layers, often with absorbable sutures for the deeper layers and non-absorbable sutures or staples for the skin.

Postoperative Care: A sterile dressing is applied, and the arm is placed in a sling for comfort.

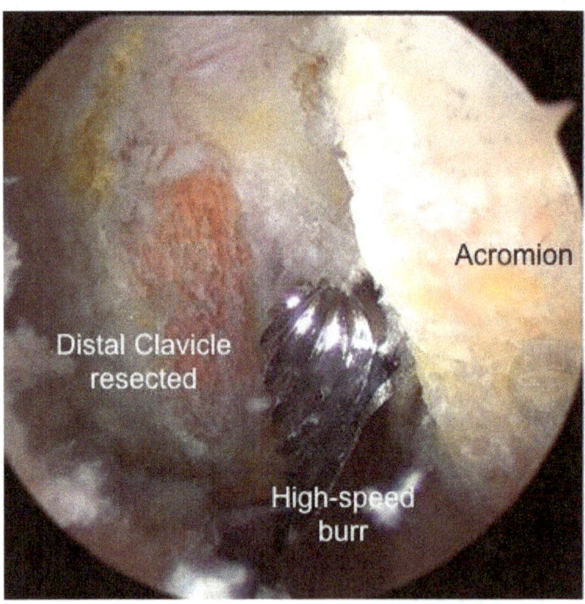

Fig. 8.4.2 Arthroscopic View of Distal Claviculectomy

ARTHROSCOPIC MUMFORD PROCEDURE

Preoperative Preparation

Anesthesia: General anesthesia is most common, but regional anesthesia can also be used.

Positioning: The patient is placed in a **Beach Chair** position. The arm is placed in a holder or allowed to hang freely for better access and visualization.

Surgical Steps

Portals and Access:

Standard arthroscopic portals are established, typically a posterior portal for viewing and an anterior portal for instrumentation.I also use a lateral portal to thin the acromion above and remove some of the clavicular end. Switching the arthroscopic view to the lateral portal is also done.

Additional portals may be made as needed to access the A-C joint. Occasionally, an anterosuperior portal directly over the joint is used in my surgeries.

JOINT VISUALIZATION AND ROUTINE INSPECTION

An arthroscope is introduced first into the glenohumeral joint for initial inspection. Then the arthroscope directed into the subacromial space to visualize the underside of the acrominon and the A-C joint.

A bursectomy is commonly performed to improve visualization and access to the joint.

DISTAL CLAVICLE RESECTION

Specialized arthroscopic instruments, such as burs, are used to resect the distal clavicle. Typically, 2 cm of the clavicle is removed. See **Fig. 8.4.1 and Fig. 8.4.2.**

The resection is performed under direct arthroscopic visualization, ensuring complete removal of the desired portion of the clavicle and smoothing of the resected surface.

Resection and thinning of the underside of the acromion is also done with the burr. This increases the space between the rotator cuff and the bony acromion. This reduces the chances of impingement or pinching laterally. The step also exposes the end of the clavicle.

After resection, the joint space is assessed to ensure adequate decompression and to confirm that no bone spurs or other impingements remain. These no contact between the clavicle and the acromion any longer.

CLOSURE:

The portals are closed with one suture or Steri-Strips, and a sterile dressing is applied.

The arm may be placed in a sling postoperatively.

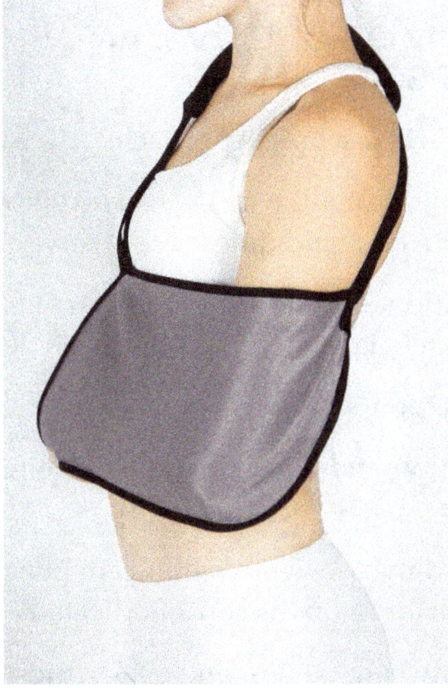

Fig. 8.4.3 Post Operative Sling

POSTOPERATIVE CARE

- **Rehabilitation:** Early passive range of motion exercises are encouraged to prevent stiffness. Strengthening exercises are gradually introduced, focusing on restoring shoulder function while protecting the AC joint.
- **Recovery:** Patients generally return to normal activities within 6-12 weeks with open procedures, depending on the extent of the procedure and physical demands.

The major advantage of an arthroscopic Mumford procedure is that there is much less trauma to the soft tissues, including the skin and muscle. The healing is much shorter, such as one to two weeks. Exercises can begin immediately, and total recovery is only about four weeks.

COMPARISON OF OPEN VS. ARTHROSCOPIC APPROACHES

Advantages of Arthroscopic Approach:

Less invasive with smaller incisions, resulting in potentially less postoperative pain and quicker recovery

Better visualization of the joint and surrounding structures which can be beneficial in complex cases.

Advantages of Open Approach:

Direct visualization and access to the A-C joint allow for more precise resection.

May be preferred in cases with significant bone deformity or in patients where arthroscopy is contraindicated.

The choice between an open or arthroscopic Mumford procedure often depends on the surgeon's experience, the patient's anatomy, and the specific pathology being treated. Both approaches have high success rates in relieving pain and restoring function in patients with AC joint pathology.

My preference when considering arthroscopic versus open A-C surgery (Mumford procedure) is definitely the arthroscopic method. This leaves no scarring other than small puncture marks. The recovery is rapid. The arthroscopic surgeon, of course, has to be familiar with how much resection he or she is going to do off the distal clavicle and the underside of the acromion. My preference is 2 cm. This arthroscopic method has been successful hundreds of times in my hands over the 43 years of practice. In my experience, it is one of the easiest shoulder procedures to learn.

9 CLAVICULAR FRACTURES

CLAVICULAR FRACTURES, COMMONLY KNOWN AS COLLARBONE fractures, are frequent injuries, especially in active individuals. They typically occur due to falls onto an outstretched hand, direct impact to the shoulder, or traumatic accidents.

CLASSIFICATION OF CLAVICLE FRACTURES:

1. Middle third: most common.
2. Distal 3rd, 15% associated with AC joints.
3. Medial 3rd least common, only 5%.
4. Displacement or angulated fractures.
5. Comminuted fractures with multiple fragments of bone.
6. Open fractures where the skin has been broken.
7. Neurovascular compromise with injury to nerves and blood vessels.

CLAVICULAR FRACTURES

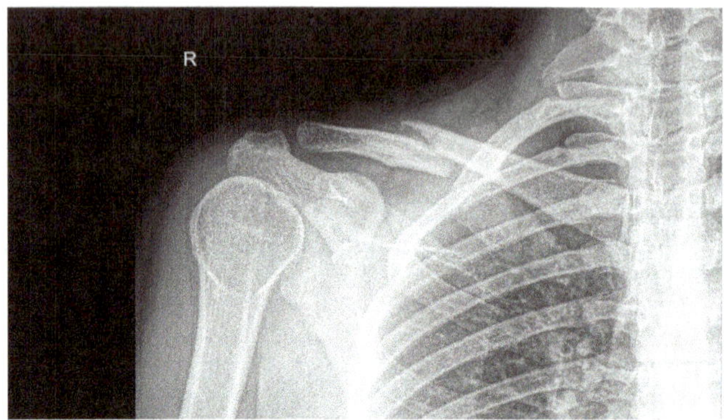

9.1.1 Mid Third Fracture of Clavicle

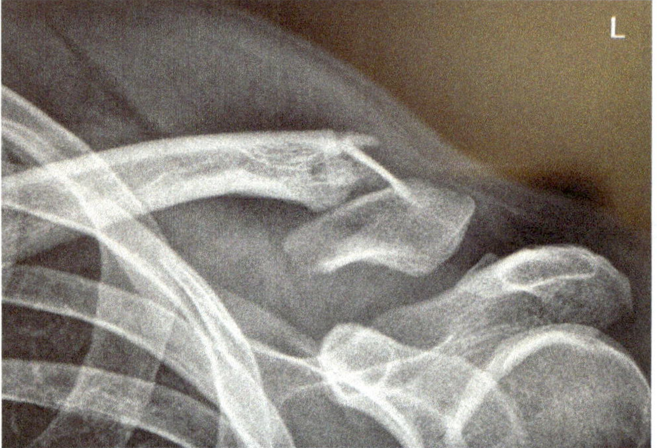

Fig. 9.1.2 Distal Third Fracture

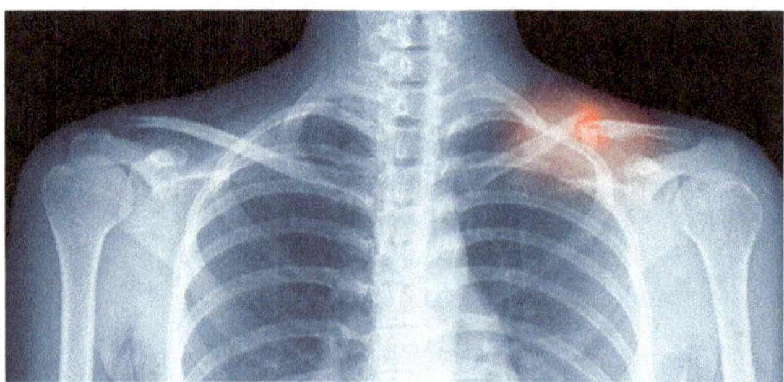

Fig. 9.1.3 Angulated Fracture

Mechanism of injury: Clavicle fractures usually occur in a fall directly onto the point of the shoulder. Also a direct blow to the clavicle from the front can fracture this bone. And then a fall onto the outstretched hand is also very common putting forces on the clavicle beyond its strength.

Symptoms: **usual symptoms** when the fracture occurs are sharp pain at the fracture site there's also a visible deformity or bump over the fracture site and then eventually swelling and bruising occur there is so much pain that there's limited shoulder movement in all case

A physical exam should include observation of the findings of swelling, tenderness, and limited motion if there is a wide displacement of the fracture. There will be an obvious deformity that demonstrates the location of the fracture.

X-rays are used to confirm the location and type of fracture; simple AP and oblique X-rays of the clavicle are all that are usually needed. In a complicated fracture, a CT scan can be helpful to create a three-dimensional impression of the situation. Only In severe fractures that involve neurological or vascular problems would an MRI be indicated.

DIAGNOSIS

After taking a thorough history and performing physical examination and X-rays we have the diagnosis of a fracture of the clavicle. There are different types of fractures of the clavicle as noted earlier and each one has to be treated differently. Some fractures are minimally displaced and can be treated conservatively in an adult. The younger the patient the more likely you can treat a clavicle conservatively, because they remodel very well.However, there are fractures that need surgical attention occasionally because of angulation, shortening, or other forms of displacement.

TREATMENT

I always start out with a conservative program including pain medication, anti-inflammatory medication, a . Rest as well as ice now in the 1st 72 hours to reduce swelling is used. If there's a minimal displacement then a continuation of the combination of a sling and a figure of eight harness is utilized. If there is too much displacement or angulation then surgery is recommended.

Physical therapy can start once the initial healing has occurred over three to four weeks. If surgery is required, usually six weeks of healing are going to be needed. Physical therapy involves range of motion and gradual strengthening. Theraband and light weights supplement manual hands-on treatment. Strengthening of the upper extremity and shoulder are emphasized.

INDICATIONS FOR SURGERY

While many clavicle fractures heal well with conservative treatment (like a sling and physical therapy), surgical intervention may be necessary in certain cases:

- Displaced fractures: Fracture ends are not aligned properly.

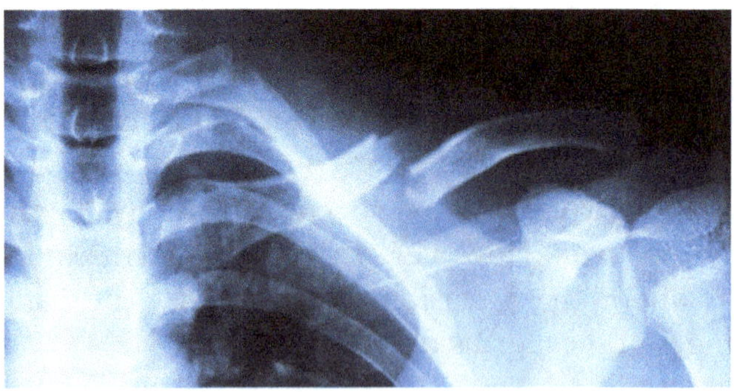

Fig. 9.2 Fracture Ends Not Aligned

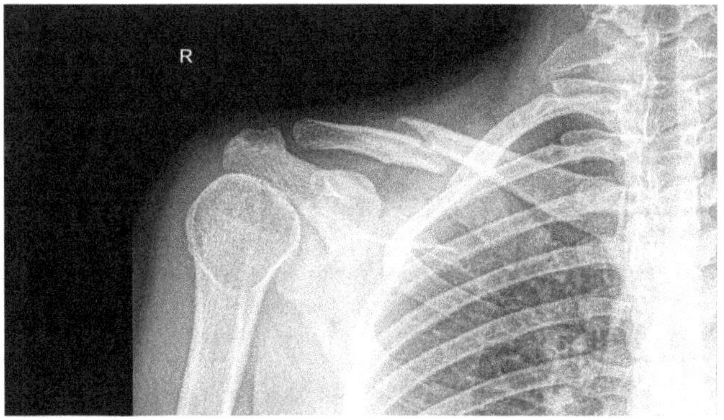

Fig. 9.3 Overlap of Bones with Shortening

DIAGNOSIS

Diagnosing a fracture of the clavicle for an orthopedic surgeon or any doctor or paramedical personnel is easy because the fracture is so obvious. However, there are different types of fractures, some requiring conservative treatment and some requiring surgical correction. The ones that have significant overlap of the fracture bones need to be lengthened and fixated with intermediary rotting or a plate. The fracture ends need to be aligned as best as possible and the pieces put back in place again as best as possible. If there is an open skin lesion where the bone was poking through, antibiotics are absolutely necessary and treatment needs to be done immediately so the infection doesn't occur. Also in some cases there are neurovascular compromised injuries to the nerves or blood vessels and this has to be addressed usually by a neurosurgeon or vascular surgeon.

Over time some fractures don't heal and one can develop nonunions where there is tissue interposing. These fractures don't heal at all or a malunion occurs where they heal non-anatomically.

And then lastly sometimes the injuries with comminution (multiple pieces) and shortening are too great to make the clavicle near anatomical. The patient is informed of this and will have to live with some limitations and disability, because of the type of fracture it was.

SURGICAL TECHNIQUES

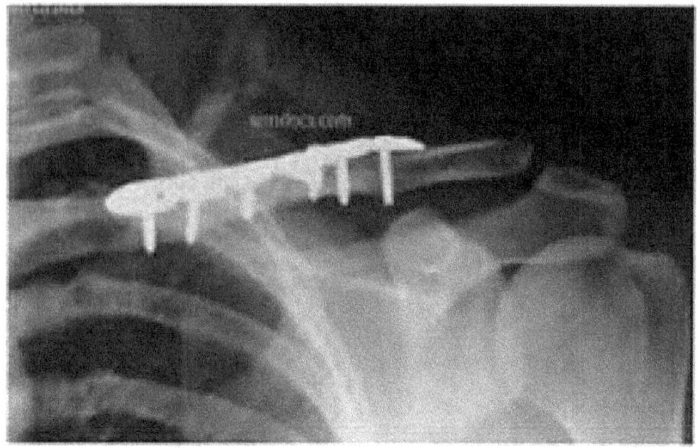

Fig. 9.4 Plating a Clavicular Fracture

OPEN REDUCTION AND INTERNAL FIXATION (ORIF):

PLATE AND SCREW FIXATION.

Incision: A horizontal incision is made over the fracture site approximately 4-5 centimeters. This gives adequate exposure to the fracture. This also allows instruments to be introduced to realign and reduce the fracture as best possible.

Reduction: The bone fragments are realigned (reduced). Grasping and moving the two main portions of the clavicle is done with specialized surgical instruments.

Fixation: Once the bone segments of the the clavicle are touching and aligned properly then fixation is next. A pre-contoured plate is placed on the superior aspect of the clavicle and secured with screws.

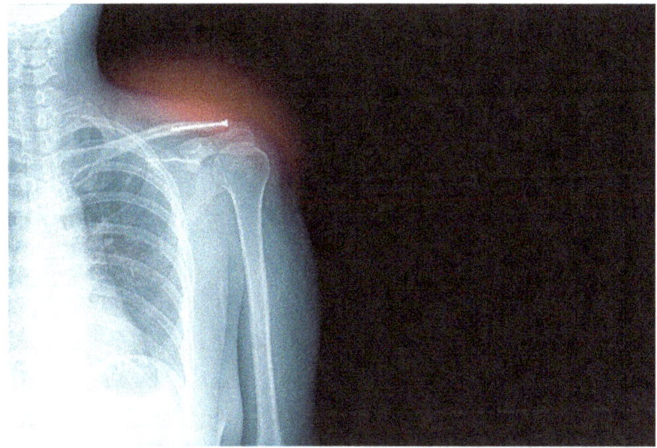

Fig. 9.5 Intramedullary Rod of Fracture

INTRAMEDULLARY FIXATION

PROCEDURE:

Incision: A small incision can be used at the fracture site in addition to the small incision at the distal clavicle. The fracture site incision is necessary to adjust the ends of the fracture while the rod is inserted across the fracture .

The purpose of the small incision at the end of the clavicle is to introduce the rod in the bone.

Reduction: The bone fragments are aligned. Reduction is the term used medically for placing the bony fragments in the most anatomical position possible.

Fixation: A flexible intramedullary rod is inserted into the medullary canal of the clavicle to stabilize the fracture. The rod or large pin is inserted at the distal end of the clavicle. At the completion of inserting the rod, an X-ray is done to confirm the proper position of the rod across the fracture site. Also the correct alignment and reduction of the fracture is noted.

External Fixation: Rarely used but may be indicated in complex cases with severe soft tissue injury.

POSTOPERATIVE CARE

Immobilization: The arm is placed in a sling for a few weeks. after approximately 3 to six weeks depending on the fixation of the fracture and instructions of the surgeon movement should begin. Movement can be assisted and should be assisted by someone for the first four to six weeks of passive motion. This is when someone else is moving the arm and the patient tells the person moving the arm how much pain they're having. There should be very little pain with this activity. After this period of six weeks, then active motion by the patient can begin without someone moving the arm.

Pain Management: Post operative pain is to be expected and pain medication that's fairly strong should be utilized. Low doses of narcotics such as oxycontin or Norco can be used very carefully. These are very addicting drugs and should be monitored closely and prescribed in very small amounts. After approximately 3 to four weeks the severe pain should be gone and over the counter NSAID's such as ibuprofen naproxen and other anti-inflammatory medication can be utilized. Acetaminophen in recommended doses should be used for pain at this time. NSAIDs and pain medication as needed.

Physical Therapy: I strongly believe that a physical therapist with knowledge of the upper extremity should be engaged, as I believe it is medically necessary. Ideally in the beginning after healing has occurred in the first three to four weeks, the physical therapist should see the patient three times per week. This frequency can be tapered down over the next several months. Gradual range-of-motion exercises followed by strengthening exercises is the program that is used. **See Chapter 7** for a detailed physical therapy program for athletes that can be applied to most patients.

CONCLUSION

Surgical management of clavicular fractures aims to restore the anatomy of the clavicle, facilitate early mobilization, and prevent complications. Each patient's case is unique, and the decision for surgery is based on the specific nature of the fracture and the patient's overall health and activity level.

10 ARTHRITIS OF THE SHOULDER JOINT

MY WORKUP AS AN ORTHOPEDIC SURGEON FOR THE DIAGNOSIS AND treatment of shoulder arthritis involves a systematic approach. The causes of shoulder arthritis can be from trauma, an inherited condition, rheumatoid arthritis, infection, and many other causes. These can end in a bone-on-bone arthritic situation of the gleno-humeral portion of the shoulder joint.

In this section, I will discuss the elements that I used in 43 years of orthopedic treatment of thousands of patients to come to an accurate diagnostic conclusion. Only after an accurate diagnosis can treatment begin. Treatment involves clinical history, physical examination, various imaging studies, and laboratory tests.

It should also be noted that I have divided up the shoulder into the glenohumeral portion of the shoulder joint and the acromioclavicular portion of the shoulder joint for a discussion of arthritis. This chapter focuses on the glenohumeral portion of the shoulder joint, and **Chapter 8** deals with the acromioclavicular joint, usually the result of injuries to the A-C joint.

CLINICAL HISTORY AND PHYSICAL EXAMINATION:

History: A good history is taken by the doctor or staff member, and this should include the duration that the patient has had the shoulder pain, such as days, weeks, months, or even years. Was there limited motion when it started, and how has it progressed?

Was there a history of trauma, such as a fall, fracture, or repetitive motion. Overuse is also a cause of micro-trauma in which, over the years, the surface of the joint wears out. Repetitive motion sports, such as pitching in baseball and passing in football, also impact hockey and football, and using a tennis racket traumatizes the joint surfaces repetitively over many years. Recently pickleball is very common in older athletes.What is the impact on daily activities from the pain and limited motion?

Pain: What was the nature of the pain (e.g., sharp, dull, constant, intermittent). Did the pain come on suddenly and severely, or was it minimal in the beginning and then gradually increased in severity. Was the pain associated with grinding, popping, or locking of the shoulder joint. Was the pain intermittent with use in certain positions or was it constant in all positions.

Grinding and a Popping Noise: An arthritic shoulder frequently has a great deal of grinding, which we call crepitus in medical terms. This is the result of very irregular surfaces that are rubbing against each other in the glenoid or cup and the humeral head or ball. Any movement causes this grinding and crepitus associated with pain usually.

Range of Motion: Is the range of motion very limiting in function such as raising the arm overhead to reach for something out of a cupboard. Is it a problem reaching in front or extending behind the shoulder in daily activities? is lifting a cup of coffee or a bottle of water painful associated with grinding and in a very limited range of motion.

Systemic Illness: Is there any presence of systemic sicknesses like fever, weight loss, or morning stiffness. These symptoms might indicate the presence of systemic arthritis conditions such as rheumatoid arthritis, gouty arthritis, psoriatic arthritis, or other conditions that may be genetic or related to infection.

PHYSICAL EXAMINATION:

Physical: In the basic physical examination, I start out with an inspection for any muscle atrophy, swelling, or unusual bony prominence, such as spurs of the A-C joint.

Palpation for tenderness, crepitus, or warmth is a very important part of the assessment. Swelling can also be felt. This would indicate a more acute condition with swelling and edema associated with possibly an acute infection or more recent acute trauma.

Range of motion: Testing (both active and passive) is extremely important in determining the severity of the arthritis. **Active** testing of range of motion indicates the patient can move the shoulder joint on his own. **Passive** range of motion indicates that the patient cannot move the arm on his/her own, and the examiner has to move the arm throughout a range of motion.

The more decreased the range of motion of the shoulder the more severe degree of joint arthritis and scarring is present. Moderate to severe limitation of motion prohibits good function and also indicates it will be difficult to easily restore the shoulder to full function.

The importance of **strength** testing of the rotator cuff muscles cannot be emphasized enough. Muscle strength will eventually be required to restore function in daily activities. From the beginning of this assessment, an estimate of the percentage of weakness is important because this will determine the time it will take to restore the strength of the shoulder muscle power. A knowledgeable physical therapist can assist the doctor in documenting the correct beginning strengths and the progress over the several weeks or months of treatment.

Specific Tests that we do as orthopedic surgeons to help determine the pathology of the shoulder. There are tests for impingement, rotator cuff tear, A-C joint arthritis pathology, and other specific tests to rule out other shoulder conditions.

IMAGING STUDIES

X-rays: Standard AP (anterior-posterior) and axillary lateral views to assess joint space narrowing, osteophytes, loose bodies of bone and calcification, subchondral sclerosis, and cysts. Previous fractures and deformities of either the glenoid, the humeral head, or AC joint are evident on these X-rays, usually.

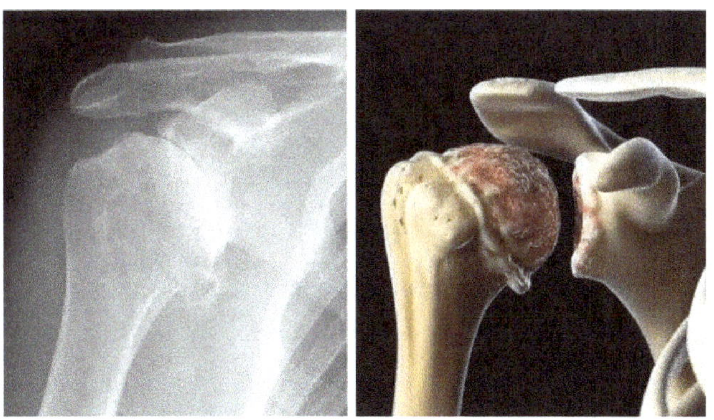

Fig. 10.1 Arthritis of the Shoulder X-Ray AP and Axillary Views

MRI. MRI is a technique that combines magnetism and ultrasound in a large tubular machine that then prints out electronically a picture of various soft tissue and bony structures in great detail. MRIs are frequently used with and without contrast Gadolinium to evaluate soft tissue structures, including the rotator cuff, labrum, cartilage, tendons, capsule, synovial fluid, and cartilaginous loose bodies. Circulation to the humeral head, as well as collapse can also be determined with this technique.

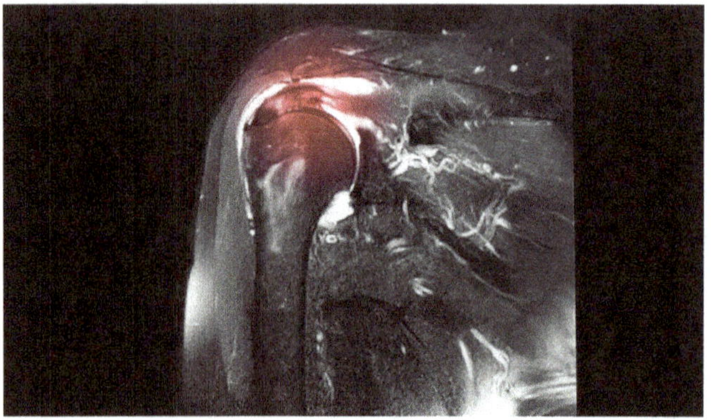

Fig. 10.2 MRI of Arthritic Shoulder with Rotator Cuff Tear

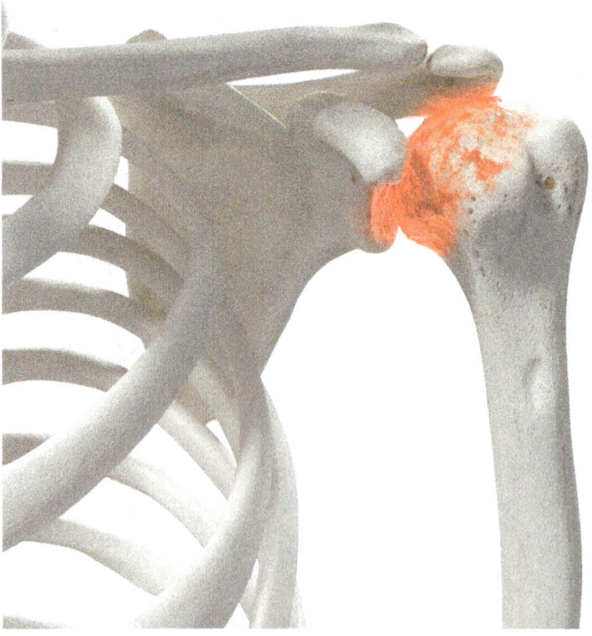

Fig. 10.3.1 Arthritis of Glenohumeral Joint

CT Scan: A CT scan is a study of detailed X-rays in slices throughout the joint area. It shows in detail osteophytes, joint space and various other pathologies in the bone mainly. I believe this study is helpful, especially in planning a surgery on an arthritic shoulder.

Ultrasound: Ultrasound is a technique that is applied to the soft tissues of the shoulder joint. In this case, various sound waves are bounced off these tissues and a picture is produced of structures that are deformed, missing, or damaged. Ultrasound is useful not only for assessing soft tissue structures but also for providing guidance for doing injections into the shoulder joint, such as in the subacromial space or in the glenohumeral portion of the shoulder joint.

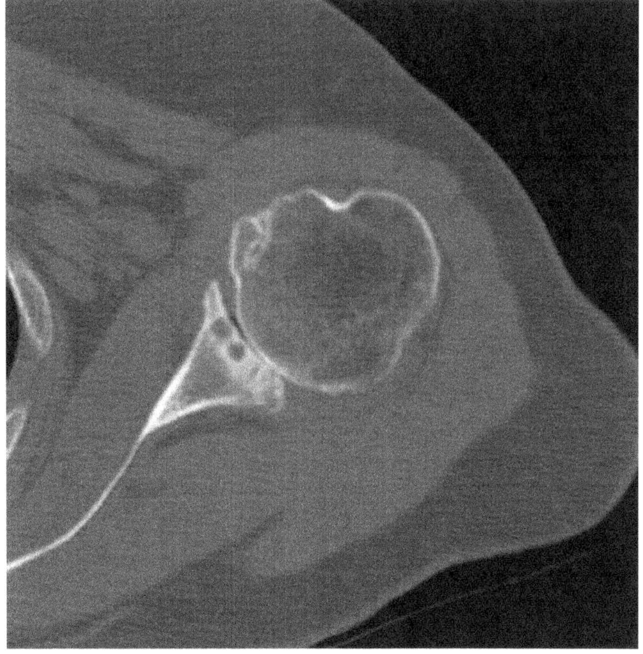

Fig. 10.3.2 CT SCAN GLENOHUMERAL

Laboratory Tests: Laboratory tests of various types are used to rule out inflammatory or infectious causes. Examples of the tests are listed below.

Complete blood count (CBC). This test measures the blood count of red cells, white cells, and platelets and differentiates the presence or absence of infection. Also, in some cases, the white and red cells can indicate various forms of arthritis.

Erythrocyte sedimentation rate (ESR) and C-reactive protein (CRP). These tests are very helpful in determining active disease when inflammatory types such as rheumatoid arthritis, psoriatic arthritis, and infectious arthritis are suspected.

Rheumatoid factor (RF) and anti-CCP antibodies are excellent and reliable tests for rheumatoid arthritis. These tests should be ordered in almost every case where there has been long-standing shoulder deterioration.

Joint aspiration and analysis if infection or crystal arthropathy is suspected. This goes beyond blood tests, but in some specific cases, it is helpful.

DIAGNOSIS

Whether there is **Post Traumatic Arthritis, Osteoarthritis, or Rheumatoid Arthritis** the end stage is treated the same. The early stages leading to end stage bone on bone arthritis can be treated initially conservatively. Gradually these conditions usually get worse over time.

TREATMENT

As always, in the treatment of an arthritic shoulder, the most conservative and the most efficient treatments to get rid of the patient's pain and improve the range of motion should be utilized. The following is simply a patient's guide to understand what types of recommendations they will encounter. They will be able to intelligently ask the treating physician/surgeon why various treatments have been recommended.

NON-SURGICAL MANAGEMENT

MEDICATIONS ARE THE FIRST LINE OF DEFENSE.

NSAIDs (Non-Steroidal Anti-Inflammatory Drugs) for pain and inflammation are the hallmarks of early treatment by conservative means for an inflamed, painful shoulder. To a certain extent, pain is also reduced by these anti-inflammatory medications. There are many choices of NSAIDs: Naproxen, Ibuprofen, Celebrex, Aleve, and other prescribed medications, as well as over-the-counter medication. These should be taken as prescribed by the physician and taken with food or an anti-acid to protect the stomach lining.

Acetaminophen is by far the most common medication used for pain relief. This drug is over-the-counter, and it gives relief for slight to moderate pain depending on the dosage and the patient. It is non-addicting. This can be taken in combination with the NSAIDs, according to instructions on the box .For example, I often will recommend two Alleve and two acetaminophen twice a day for moderate pain.

In patients with moderate to severe pain that is constant and unrelenting, a **Pain Management Physician** should play a role. If activities of daily living, as well as sleep, are very significantly affected, it is my recommendation that a stronger pain medication should be prescribed. There are safe ways to prescribe Tramadol, Oxycontin, Norco, and others controlled drugs in very low dosages that will relieve pain.

In probably 1 out of 10 patients, there is a risk of addiction. Caution has to be used in prescribing narcotics as well as their utilization. In my opinion, **co-operation** between the patient, the orthopedic surgeon, and the pain management doctor is required.

INJECTIONS

Intra-articular corticosteroid injections for acute exacerbations are indispensable. Since 1976, when I started my orthopedic practice, I have utilized these injections.

My injections are a mixture of 1 CC/40mg Depo-medrol, 3 CCs of Lidocaine 1.0%, and 3 CCs of Marcaine 0.5%. This is injected sterility, usually into the subacromial space or into the glenohumeral portion of the shoulder joint.

These can also be used as **trigger point injections** in muscles around the shoulder. Within minutes, the pain is relieved, and the long-acting anesthetic gives relief for about 14 hours. In my experience, the Depo-medrol component will reduce inflammation for months at a time. There is minimal risk with these injections.

There can be a rare infection that can be treated with antibiotics. It should be noted that a variety of cortisone derivatives, as well as anesthetic choices can be used for the injections. Also, if a physician feels more comfortable using ultrasound to locate the subacromial joint and the glenohumeral joint, this can be done in an operating room, but usually, this can be done in the office setting without ultrasound.

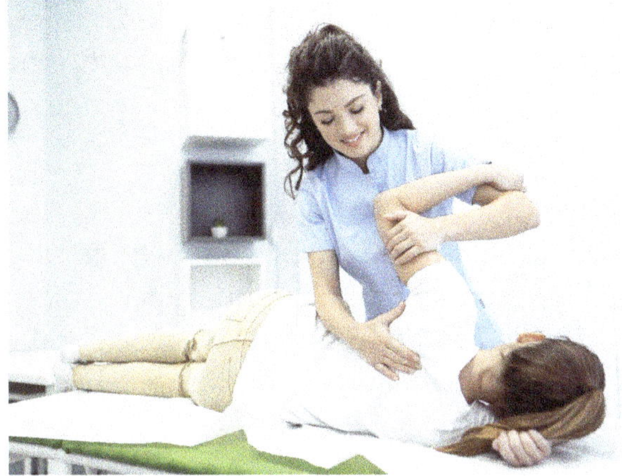

Fig 10.4 Range of Motion Exercise

PHYSICAL THERAPY

Range of motion (ROM) exercises to maintain joint mobility can be painful in an arthritic shoulder and are usually associated with a great deal of grinding, but they should be done anyway. If ROM is not maintained, the success of any treatment in an arthritic shoulder is doomed. The patient will get a frozen shoulder that will be useless and extremely stiff.

Strengthening exercises for the shoulder muscles are necessary. Using lightweights and daily exercises, doing only 10 or 20 reps in each direction of flexion, extension, and abduction will maintain the strength of the shoulder muscles and functional use of the entire arm. If the deltoid, biceps, or triceps muscles cannot move the shoulder even in spite of a rotator cuff tear or arthritis, then once again, this shoulder will be useless. This is why it is so important to use lightweight weights and do daily exercise to strengthen the shoulder muscles, even though it's probably going to be painful.

Heat/cold therapy and ultrasound treatments have been utilized to alleviate some of the pain in the shoulder area. Each person has a unique response, in my opinion, to the heat to ease pain at rest. Cold is better used for 15 to 20 minutes after an exercise program to reduce swelling. Ultrasound and thumper devices applied to the muscle seem to alleviate some of the pain as well.

Activity Modification Avoiding activities that exacerbate symptoms, such as overhead use or repetitive use in the overhead position, is discouraged. This type of activity will aggravate an arthritic condition and also cause a great deal of pain. Painful movements should be restricted to physical therapy with the guidance of a therapist at that time.

Use of assistive devices or braces for the shoulder is limited because the shoulder is not a weight-bearing joint that usually requires a cane or any other type of device such as that. However, there is a shoulder brace that pulls the shoulder somewhat tighter if it is loose and painful. These are available commercially on the Internet or through an orthopedic office.

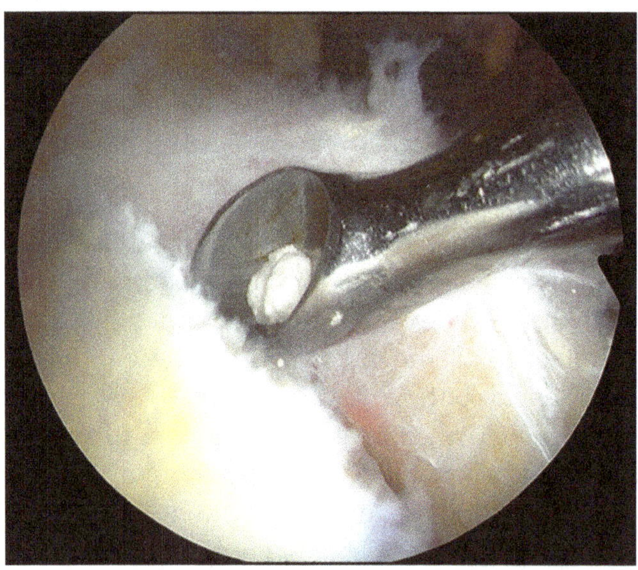

Fig. 10.5 Arthroscopic Debridement of Arthritic Joint

SURGICAL MANAGEMENT:

Shoulder Arthroscopy A minimally invasive procedure to debride the joint, remove loose bodies, or perform synovectomy is commonly done. This requires three small punctures in the skin of the shoulder. **See Fig. 2.6**

A telescope called an arthroscope is inserted into one of the punctures, while operating instruments to vacuum, grasp, and cut are inserted into the other punctures. A power shaver, cutter, and cautery are introduced as well to perform synovectomy. See **Fig.. 2.4.1** Synovectomy removes the painful lining of the joint that produces excessive joint fluid. This procedure is done under general anesthesia. The risks are minimal. Failure to achieve a desired result and infection are the main infrequent complications.

JOINT IMPLANT SURGERY

Implants When an arthritic shoulder deteriorates at the end stage of a very painful bone on bone, it is time to consider an **Implant** . There are three types of implants. In the first type **Hemiarthroplasty** the humeral head is replaced only. In the second type both the humeral head and the glenoid are replaced. The third type also replaces the humeral head and glenoid, but not anatomically.

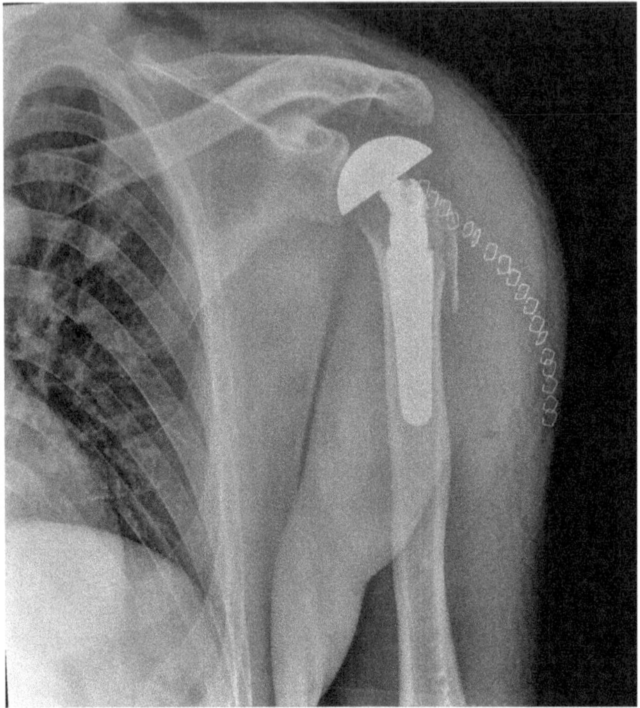

Fig. 10.6 Hemiarthroplasty of the Shoulder

Hemiarthroplasty This procedure involves the replacement of the humeral Head alone. Replacing the humeral head only in an arthritic shoulder generally has a good success rate, but it varies based on several factors. These include the underlying cause of the arthritis, the patient's age, activity level, and overall health. These are some key points regarding its success rate.

This procedure is also frequently used in three-part and four-part fractures of the humeral head with older soft bone. The head can't be repaired so it is replaced.

HEMI-ARTHROPLASTY PROCEDURE

Here's a step-by-step description of the procedure:

Preoperative Preparation: The patient undergoes a thorough preoperative medical and cardiac evaluation, including EKG and chest X-ray, as well as imaging studies like shoulder X-rays, CT scans, or MRIs to assess the condition of the shoulder joint.

The patient is given anesthesia, usually general anesthesia or a regional block, to numb the shoulder area.

Incision and Exposure: A surgical incision is made anteriorly over the shoulder joint, typically through the deltopectoral groove (between the deltoid and pectoral muscles).

The surgeon carefully dissects through the soft tissues to expose the shoulder joint, taking care to protect the surrounding nerves and blood vessels.

Removal of the Humeral Head: The humeral head is dislocated from the glenoid (socket) to gain better access.

The damaged or arthritic humeral head is removed using specialized surgical instruments.

Preparation of the Humeral Shaft: The humeral shaft (the long bone extending from the shoulder to the elbow) is prepared to receive the prosthetic implant.

The bone is shaped and reamed on the inside of this tubular bone to create a precise fit for the prosthesis.

Insertion of the Prosthesis: A metal or ceramic prosthetic Humeral Head is inserted into the prepared humeral shaft.

The prosthesis is secured using either cemented or uncemented techniques, depending on the patient's bone quality and the surgeon's preference.

Reattachment of Soft Tissues: The surgeon reattaches the soft tissues, including the rotator cuff tendons and muscles to ensure proper stability and function of the shoulder joint.

The joint is tested for range of motion and stability

Closure: The surgical incision is closed in layers using sutures or staples.

A sterile dressing is applied to the wound.

Postoperative Care: The patient is taken to the recovery room and monitored as the anesthesia wears off.

Pain management, antibiotics, and blood clot prevention measures are initiated.

Once home or in an extended care facility, the patient undergoes a rehabilitation program involving physical therapy to regain shoulder strength and mobility.

Hemiarthroplasty is often indicated when the glenoid (socket) is relatively healthy and only the humeral head is severely damaged. It can provide significant pain relief and improve shoulder function, although the outcomes may vary depending on the underlying condition and the patient's overall health.

Pain Relief and Function: Hemiarthroplasty often provides significant pain relief and improved shoulder function. Many patients experience good to excellent outcomes, particularly in terms of pain reduction.

Durability: The longevity of a hemiarthroplasty can vary. Studies have shown that many patients still have a well-functioning implant 10-15 years post-surgery. However, younger and more active patients might experience wear and tear sooner.

Revision Rates: The revision rate for hemiarthroplasty is generally higher than for total shoulder arthroplasty (TSA). Patients might eventually require a conversion to TSA if the glenoid (shoulder socket) becomes increasingly arthritic.

Complications: As with any surgery, complications can occur, including infection, nerve injury, fracture, or problems with the implant.

Patient Satisfaction: Most patients report high levels of satisfaction with their outcomes, especially in terms of pain relief. However, the satisfaction rates might be slightly lower compared to those of total shoulder arthroplasty.

Comparison with TSA: Total shoulder arthroplasty, which replaces both the humeral head and the glenoid, often shows better outcomes in terms of pain relief, function, and longevity compared to hemiarthroplasty.

TOTAL SHOULDER ARTHROPLASTY (TSA):

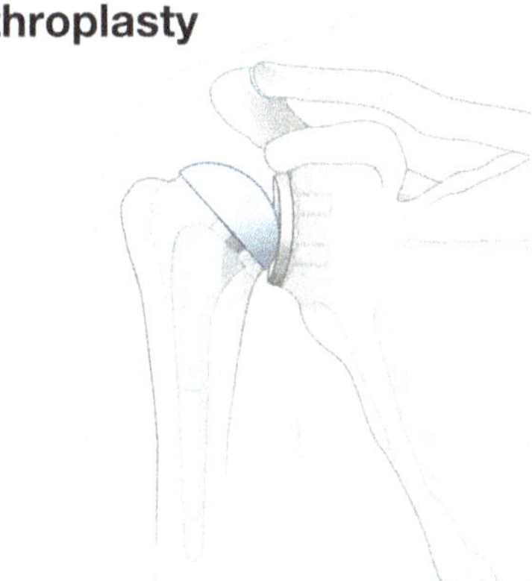

Fig.10.7 Total Shoulder Arthroplasty

Total shoulder arthroplasty (TSA), also known as shoulder replacement surgery, is performed to relieve pain and restore function in patients with severe shoulder joint arthritis or damage. Here's a step-by-step description of the procedure:

PREOPERATIVE PREPARATION

Anesthesia The patient is given general anesthesia or a regional nerve block to ensure they are pain-free and unconscious during the procedure.

Positioning The patient is placed in a semi-reclining position, often referred to as the **Beach Chair** position, to provide the surgeon with optimal access to the shoulder joint.

SURGICAL PROCEDURE

Incision A deltopectoral incision is made from just above the clavicle down to the deltoid muscle. This allows access to the shoulder joint without cutting through major muscles.

Exposure The deltoid and pectoral muscles are carefully separated. The cephalic vein is usually retracted laterally or medially to protect it during the procedure.

Dissection The subscapularis tendon is released or split to expose the joint capsule. The joint capsule is then opened to reveal the humeral head.

Humeral Head Resection The humeral head is dislocated from the glenoid. The humeral head is then cut off using a surgical saw, and the humeral canal is prepared to receive the prosthetic stem. This involves reaming the canal to the appropriate size and shape.

Glenoid Preparation: The glenoid cavity is prepared by removing any remaining cartilage and shaping the bone to fit the glenoid component. A small amount of bone may be removed to create a flat surface.

IMPLANT PLACEMENT:

Humeral Component: The humeral stem is inserted into the humeral canal, and the appropriate-sized humeral head component is attached to the stem.

Glenoid Component: The glenoid component is cemented or press-fitted into the prepared glenoid cavity.

Reduction and Stability: The humeral head component is reduced into the glenoid component to ensure proper fit and stability. The range of motion and stability of the joint are checked to ensure proper alignment and function.

Closure: The subscapularis tendon is repaired, and the muscles and tissues are meticulously closed in layers. Drains may be placed to remove excess fluid from the surgical site.

Wound Closure: The skin is closed using sutures or staples, and a sterile dressing is applied.

POSTOPERATIVE CARE

Recovery: The patient is taken to the recovery room and monitored until the anesthesia wears off. Pain management is initiated.

Immobilization: The arm is typically placed in a sling to immobilize the shoulder and allow for initial healing.

Rehabilitation: Physical therapy begins soon after surgery to restore range of motion and strengthen the shoulder muscles. At home or in a nursing facility, rehabilitation is a crucial part of the recovery process and continues for several months. At first, range of motion exercises are started gently, then rapidly progress to full range of motion depending on the level of pain. My experience is that strong pain medication is required for about two months.

FOLLOW-UP

Regular follow-up appointments weekly are necessary to monitor the healing process, check the function of the prosthetic components, and ensure the patient is progressing well with rehabilitation.

Total Shoulder Arthroplasty is a complex procedure, but it can provide significant pain relief and improve the quality of life for patients with severe shoulder conditions.

The success rate of shoulder **TSA** can vary based on various factors, such as the patient's age, the severity of the condition, surgical technique, postoperative care, and the experience of the surgeon. Here is an overview of the success rates and outcomes for total shoulder arthroplasty TSA.

TSA is typically performed for patients with severe osteoarthritis, rheumatoid arthritis, or post-traumatic arthritis. The success rates for TSA are generally high.

Pain relief and functional improvement: Most patients experience significant pain relief and improved shoulder function after a healing period of several weeks.

Patient satisfaction: Patient satisfaction is reported to be around 90 to 95%. This includes range of motion, pain relief, and functional improvement.

Survivorship: The survivorship of the prosthetic joint rates are approximately 90 to 95% at 10 years; and around 85% at 20 years.

There is a revision rate that occurs in total shoulders and this revision rate depends upon unused time as well as some complications. Some complications that occur are infection, prosthetic loosening, rotator cuff tears, and periprosthetic fractures. All of these revisions are possible, and improvement can be achieved for the patient.

Reverse Total Shoulder Arthroplasty (RTSA): Used in cases with rotator cuff absence from severe tearing, severe joint damage, post-traumatic arthritis, and failed previous shoulder surgery.

SURGICAL PROCEDURE.

PREOPERATIVE PREPARATION

Evaluation and Planning: Detailed patient history and physical examination.

Imaging studies (X-rays, CT scans, or MRIs) to assess the condition of the shoulder.

Preoperative planning with templating software to determine the correct size and positioning of implants.

Anesthesia: General anesthesia or regional nerve block.

SURGICAL PROCEDURE

Patient Positioning: The patient is positioned in a Beach Chair position, semi-upright, with the head elevated.

Incision: A deltopectoral or superior approach is commonly used. An incision is made over the shoulder joint.

Exposure: Dissection through the deltoid and pectoral muscles to expose the shoulder joint.

Careful identification and protection of the axillary nerve.

Glenoid Preparation: The glenoid cavity (socket of the shoulder blade) is exposed.

Removal of any remaining cartilage and preparation of the bone surface.

Placement of the baseplate and fixation with screws into the glenoid bone.

Humeral Preparation: Exposure of the proximal humerus (upper arm bone).

Removal of the humeral head and preparation of the humeral canal.

Placement of the humeral stem into the canal, cemented or press-fit.

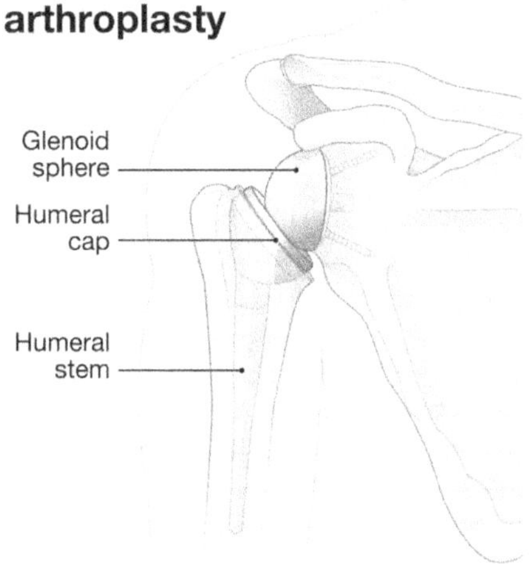

Fig. 10.8 Reverse total Shoulder Arthroplasty

Implantation: Attachment of the glenosphere (ball component) to the baseplate on the Glenoid.

Placement of the polyethylene cup (socket) onto the Humeral stem.

Reduction: The new ball (glenosphere) and socket (polyethylene cup) components are articulated to restore shoulder function.

Closure: Layered closure of the soft tissues and skin.

Placement of a drain, if necessary.

POSTOPERATIVE CARE

Recovery: Monitoring in the recovery room until stable.

Pain management with medications.

Initial immobilization of the shoulder with a sling or brace.

Rehabilitation: Physical therapy to regain motion and strength.

Gradual progression of activities under the guidance of a physical therapist.

Follow-Up: Regular follow-up visits weekly to monitor healing and implant position.

POTENTIAL COMPLICATIONS

- Infection
- Nerve injury
- Dislocation of the implant
- Fracture
- Loosening of the implant over time

RTSA can significantly improve shoulder function and reduce pain in patients with complex shoulder conditions that are not amenable to other treatments.

Follow-Up and Rehabilitation: Regular follow-up to monitor the progression of the disease and respond to treatment.

Postoperative rehabilitation to ensure optimal recovery and function after surgery.

ADDITIONAL CONSIDERATIONS

Patient Education: Informing patients about the nature of the disease, treatment options, and realistic outcomes.

Multidisciplinary Approach: Collaboration with rheumatologists, physical therapists, and pain specialists as needed.

Lifestyle Modifications: Encouraging weight management, healthy diet, and low-impact exercises to support joint health.

11 HUMERAL HEAD FRACTURES

Proximal Humeral fractures (breaks) are common, especially among the elderly. A fall on an outstretched arm or direct trauma to the shoulder is the most frequent cause of this injury. The proximal humerus bone includes the humeral head, anatomical neck, surgical neck, and the greater and lesser tuberosities.

HISTORY AND SYMPTOMS

Patients typically present with severe pain around the shoulder, soft tissue swelling,bruising, and limited movement. Sometimes there is a visible deformity.

SPECIAL STUDIES

Diagnosis is confirmed through imaging studies.

X-rays:First initial studies, including AP, lateral, and axillary views of the shoulder are extremely necessary. X-rays show the bones, fractures, and relationships of different fragments to each other.

CT scan: For more complex fractures or when surgical planning is needed, the CT scan gives a 3- dimensional view of the bony fracture fragments and their orientation.

MRI: Sometimes used to evaluate associated soft tissue injuries such as rotator cuff tear or damage to the neurovascular structures.

DIAGNOSIS

Almost all of the **Humeral Head Fractures** are caused by falls or severe direct impact such as in a car accident. These fractures are described in four parts.

The treatment approach depends on the classification of the Humeral Head fractures and the patient.

The Neer classification system is commonly used to describe these fractures. It is based on the number of fracture parts, displacement, and angulation.

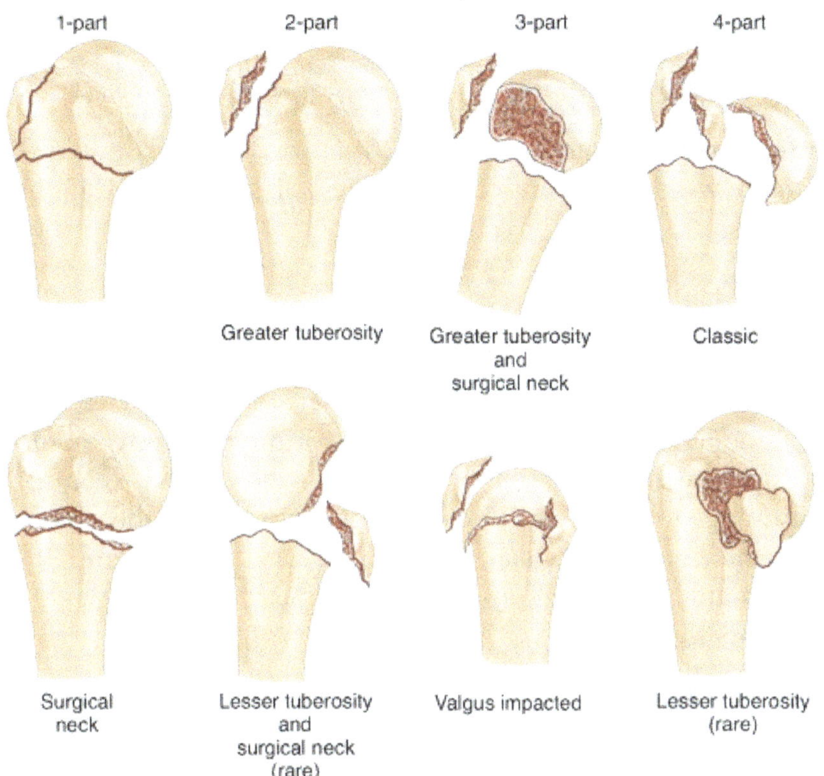

Fig. 11.1 Neer Classification of Humeral Head Fractures

One-part fracture: No significant displacement or angulation (<1 cm and <45 degrees, respectively).

Two-part fracture: Displacement of one fragment relative to the others.

Three-part fracture: Involves the surgical neck and one tubercle.

Four-part fracture: Involves the surgical neck, both tubercles and the humeral head.

TREATMENT

Non-Surgical Treatment

Indications: Minimally displaced fractures (one-part fractures), patients with significant comorbidities, or low-demand elderly patients.

Methods:

Immobilization: Using a sling or shoulder immobilizer for 2-3 weeks

Will alleviate acute pain and prevent additional movement of the fracture fragments. after the third week if the fracture is beginning to heal and no surgery was done then gentle movement can be started. If surgery was done then consultation with the surgeon is necessary to know when to move his shoulder.

Pain management: the most common treatments for pain inflammation in a fracture of the shoulder would be the NSAID's for the inflammation and acetaminophen for the pain. If these are not sufficient to alleviate the pain then opioids such as oxycontin or Norco in low doses can be prescribed and used with caution.

Physical therapy: after the period of uh two to three weeks of immobilization uh if no surgery has been done a gentle physical therapy can begin.Early passive range-of-motion exercises, progressing to active and strengthening exercises are done at a rate that is dependent on the patient's pain tolerance. Shoulder fractures notoriously hurt a great deal and a therapist that's gentle but persistent can achieve almost a full range of motion over a period of two to three months.

SURGICAL TREATMENT

Indications: in cases where the fractures are complicated and there are displaced fragments three parts or four part fractures occasionally with vascular compromise surgery is indicated. In a younger patient open reduction internal fixation or pins can be utilized. In older patients the bone is usually soft or brittle and is difficult to use fixation but it should be tried to stabilize these fractures as best as possible. We're discussing below several methods of fracture fixation.

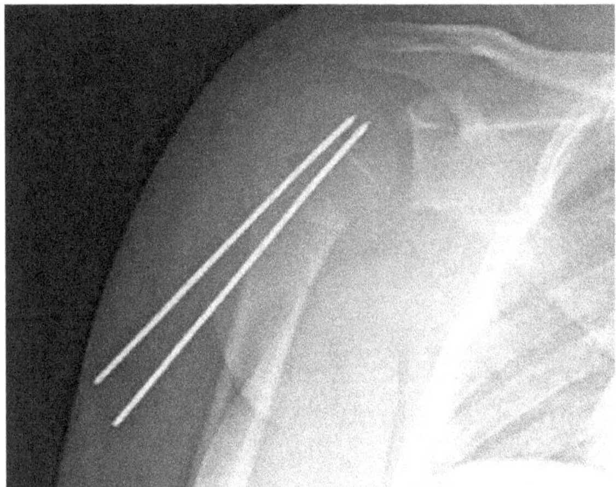

Post-operative X-ray following pediatric percutaneous pinning procedure (pins to be removed once initial healing is completed at about three weeks)

Fig. 11.2 Percutaneous Pinning

SURGICAL METHODS:

Closed reduction and percutaneous pinning: this technique can be used for less complex fractures and especially in young patients with good strong bone. This procedure is done using an X-ray image intensifier for the localization of the fracture fragments and the alignment of the pins. A motorized power drill is used to place the pins efficiently and accurately.

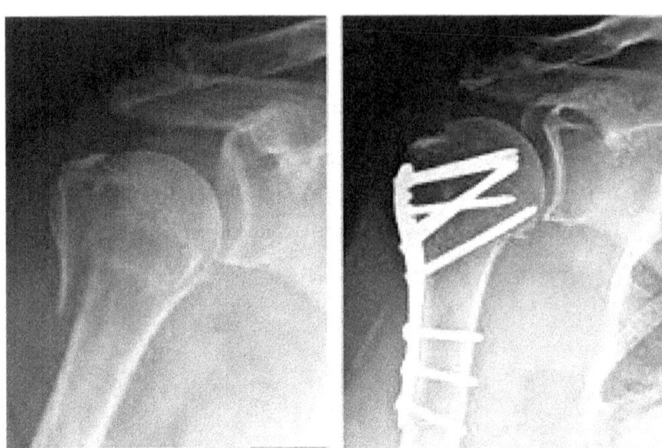

Fig.11.3 Open Reduction Internal Fixation

Open reduction and internal fixation (ORIF): Using plates and screws, often for displaced two-part, three-part, and some four-part fractures. This involves a wide open exposure moving skin and muscles with a direct visualization of the fracture fragments and their displacement. Plates and screws, and sometimes rods, are utilized to secure these fragments in as good a position as possible.

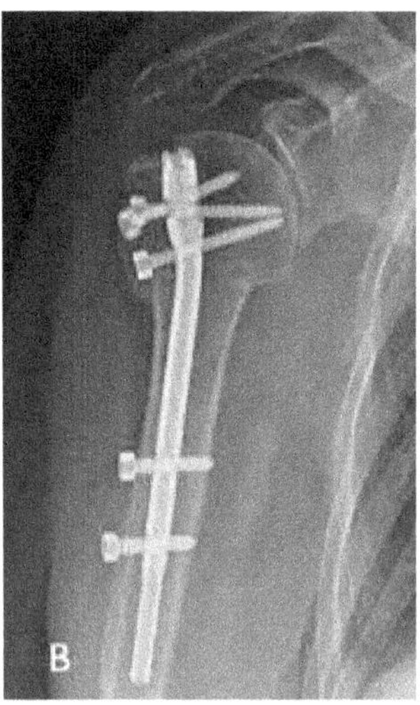

Fig. 11.4 Intramedullary Nailing

Intramedullary nailing: For selected fractures involving the surgical neck, a metal rod is introduced through the humeral head down into the shaft of the humerus, thus securing the bone. This is analogous to attaching an ice cream to a cone in an anatomical position. Once again the X-ray image intensifier is utilized in this case.

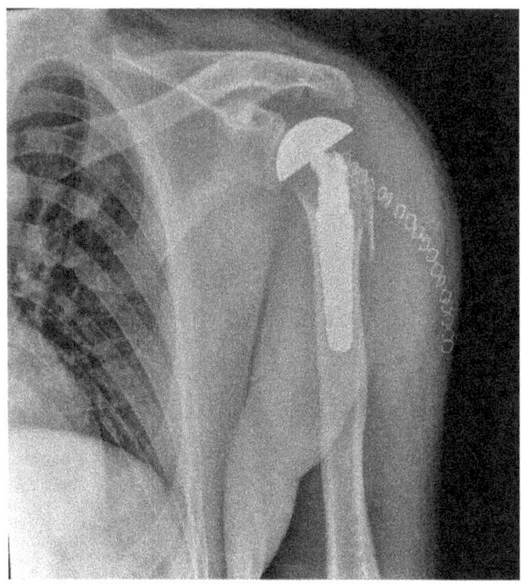

Fig. 11.5 Hemiarthroplasty

Hemiarthroplasty: Replacement of the humeral head, typically for four-part fractures or in cases with head comminution. This is done because the fragments are so small and fragile and have lost their blood supply that healing would be very difficult and not anatomical. A metal ball with a stem that goes down into the humeral shaft is placed by the surgeon carefully to provide a functional and relatively painless result for the patient.**See Chapter 10.**

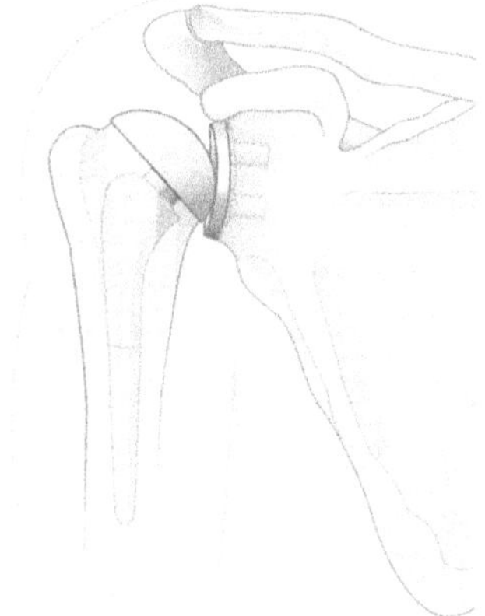

Fig. 11.6 Total Shoulder

Total shoulder arthroplasty (TSA), also known as shoulder replacement surgery, is performed to relieve pain and restore function in patients with severe shoulder joint arthritis or damage. There is a requirement that the patient still has a rotator cuff intact to do this procedure. It is not unusual in my experience that humeral head fractures occur in patients with arthritic shoulders. Depending on the patient's anticipated level of activity after recovery, a TSA is a good choice. Here's a step-by-step description of the procedure:

PREOPERATIVE PREPARATION

Anesthesia: The patient is given general anesthesia or a regional nerve block to ensure they are pain-free and unconscious during the procedure.

Positioning: The patient is placed in a semi-reclining position, often referred to as the **Beach Chair** position, to provide the surgeon with optimal access to the shoulder joint.

SURGICAL PROCEDURE

Incision: A deltopectoral incision is made from just above the clavicle down to the deltoid muscle. This allows access to the shoulder joint without cutting through major muscles.

Exposure: The deltoid and pectoral muscles are carefully separated. The cephalic vein is usually retracted laterally or medially to protect it during the procedure.

Dissection: The subscapularis tendon is released or split to expose the joint capsule. The joint capsule is then opened to reveal the humeral head.

Humeral Head Resection: The humeral head is dislocated from the glenoid. The humeral head is then cut off using a surgical saw, and the humeral canal is prepared to receive the prosthetic stem. This involves reaming the canal to the appropriate size and shape.

Glenoid Preparation: The glenoid cavity is prepared by removing any remaining cartilage and shaping the bone to fit the glenoid component. A small amount of bone may be removed to create a flat surface.

Implant Placement:

Humeral Component: The humeral stem is inserted into the humeral canal, and the appropriate-sized humeral head component is attached to the stem.

Glenoid Component: The glenoid component is cemented or press-fitted into the prepared glenoid cavity.

Reduction and Stability: The humeral head component is reduced into the glenoid component to ensure proper fit and stability. The range of motion and stability of the joint are checked to ensure proper alignment and function.

Closure: The subscapularis tendon is repaired, and the muscles and tissues are meticulously closed in layers. Drains may be placed to remove excess fluid from the surgical site.

Wound Closure: The skin is closed using sutures or staples, and a sterile dressing is applied.

POSTOPERATIVE CARE

Recovery: The patient is taken to the recovery room and monitored until the anesthesia wears off. Pain management is initiated.

Immobilization: The arm is typically placed in a sling to immobilize the shoulder and allow for initial healing.

Rehabilitation: Physical therapy begins soon after surgery to restore range of motion and strengthen the shoulder muscles. Rehabilitation is a crucial part of the recovery process and continues for several months. a sling is worn as needed to alleviate pain and to protect the surgery. depending on the patient's tolerance for pain the sling can be worn up to three or four months but the patient should be encouraged to eliminate the sling as much as possible or as early as possible.

FOLLOW-UP

Regular follow-up appointments are necessary to monitor the healing process, check the function of the prosthetic components, and ensure the patient is progressing well with rehabilitation. not only physical examination and history are taken with each visit but X-rays are needed to determine the position of the implants.

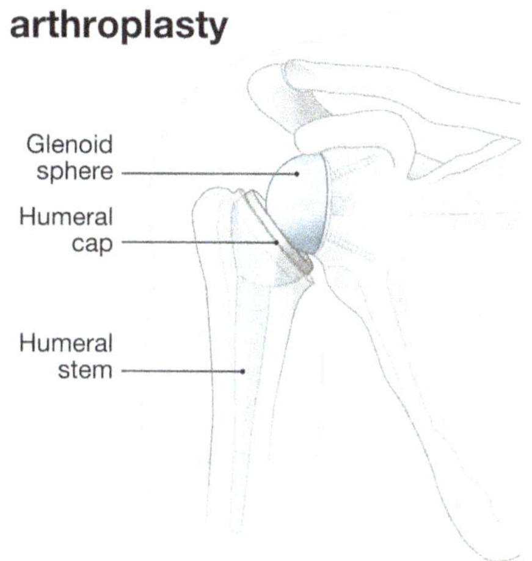

Fig. 11.7 Reverse Total Shoulder Arthroplasty

Reverse Total Shoulder Arthroplasty: Increasingly used for complex fractures, especially in older adults with poor bone quality or pre-existing rotator cuff pathology. This involves extensive detailed surgical replacement of the humeral ahead as well as the glenoid.

The surgical procedure in detail is discussed specifically in **Chapter 10**.

POSTOPERATIVE CARE

Basically, for all of the surgical treatments, the postoperative care is essentially the same.

Immobilization: Initially, this is done during surgery after surgical dressings are applied to the wound. A sling or shoulder immobilizer is utilized and worn for the next four to six weeks. Dressing changes, of course, are done over those four to six weeks by a nurse during doctor's office visits weekly.

Pain management: Surgical pain is usually very intense for the first 48 to 72 hours. After that, this pain usually reduces to a moderate level. We use a zero to 10 scale, with 10 being the most pain and zero is no pain. In my experience with patients most postoperative patients have nine or ten level pain. After the first 72 hours, it drops to about a 7 or 6 for about two weeks. Then, usually, it's in the 2 to 3 range thereafter. In some patients, pain can persist on a chronic basis and require a Pain Management Specialist to help them live with the pain in their shoulder.

Rehabilitation: Gradual physical therapy is started with **passive motion**. This is where the physical therapist lifts the arm in various directions for the patient to regain the range of motion. Next, the patient is encouraged to move their arm on their own with the assistance of the physical therapist. This is called active assist.

Therapy then progresses to **active motion** by the patient themselves in a strengthening program starting with very small weights such as one pound. Strengthening exercises are done in all directions.

Full range of motion is rarely achieved with the reverse shoulder implant.

FOLLOW-UP

Regular follow-up appointments weekly are necessary to monitor the healing process, check the function of the prosthetic components, and ensure the patient is progressing well with rehabilitation. patients should expect a physical examination of the shoulder wound check as well as an X-ray of the implant.

COMPLICATIONS

Complications can include:

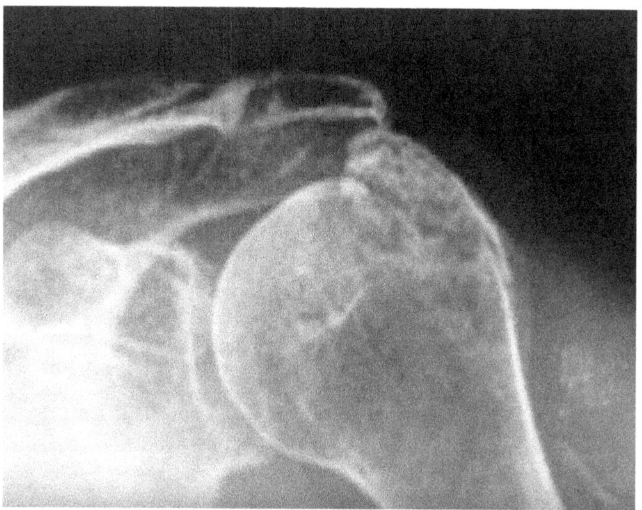

Fig. 11.8 Malunion of Humeral Head Fracture

COMPLICATIONS

Complications can include nonunion a bacterial necrosis as well as infection and failure to accomplish the goal of a painless full range of motion.

Nonunion occurs when the bones fail to mend bone to bone. **Malunion** is when the bones heal out of position and with deformity. Both of these types of failures to unite in a relatively anatomical position may cause problems for the patient. In particular, the nonunion can cause chronic pain. Each case is very individualized in terms of an attempted solution.

Avascular Necrosis is another complication of fractures of the Humeral Head. The fragments that are broken lose their blood supply and the bone dies.

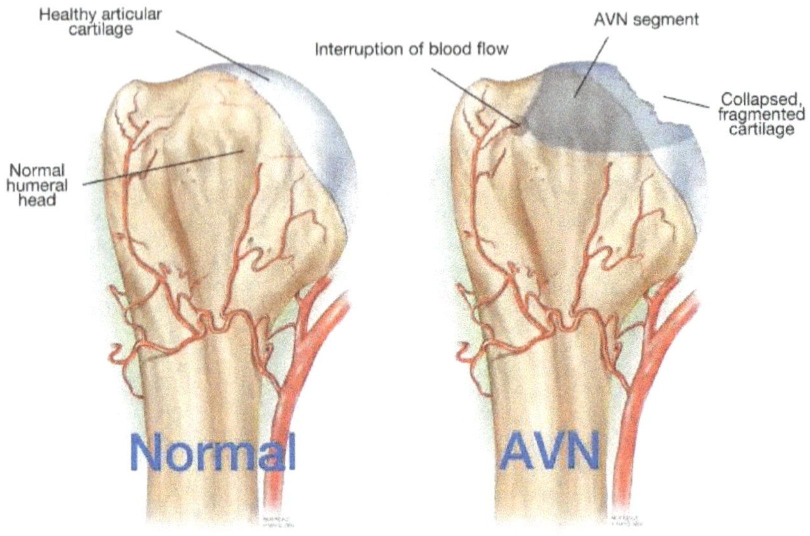

Fig. 11.9 Avascular Necrosis of Humeral Head

Avascular necrosis of the humeral head, especially in four-part fractures. The term avascular literally means without blood supply. This indicates that the bone fragment that is disconnected in a 4 part fracture from any muscle or soft tissue loses its blood supply at the time of the fracture and does not heal. This bone eventually dies and causes deformity and pain. Usually, the solution is to do a **Hemiarthroplasty** of the shoulder, replacing the humeral head or performing a **Total Shoulder**, replacing the humeral head and the glenoid. Both of these surgical procedures are described in detail in chapter 10. If there is a very badly torn rotator cuff that cannot be repaired then a **Reverse Total shoulder** is recommended.

Nerve injury can occur particularly to the axillary nerve. It may be damaged in the original fracture injury. Also, occasionally, the axillary nerve is damaged during surgery. There is no good solution for a damaged axillary nerve that supplies the motor function of the deltoid muscle.

Shoulder stiffness and reduced range of motion are a common outcome of severe humeral head fractures. Physical therapy and **Pain Management** combined are the only solutions for this type of problem. Many times, in spite of a limited range of motion and stiffness, function is preserved, so ideally, the patient can carry on their normal activities of daily living despite their limitations in motion.

Infection is almost always the result of surgical contamination. Occasionally, a patient has an infection elsewhere in their body at the time of the accident, and the infection spreads through the bloodstream to the shoulder. The treatment for this type of infection is antibiotics IV. A single antibiotic or antibiotics in combination may be required to cure this type of infection. There is always a risk of osteomyelitis (bone infection), which can be extremely difficult to treat.

Chronic Pain Syndrome occasionally develops. There are various causes of this, ranging from nonunion to infection to nerve involvement from deep scarring. The specialty of **Pain Management** is consulted, and it is important in the treatment of a patient with this condition.

PROGNOSIS

The prognosis varies based on the severity of the fracture and the patient's adherence to rehabilitation. Generally, non-displaced fractures have a good prognosis with conservative treatment, while displaced fractures may have variable outcomes depending on the surgical success, postoperative rehabilitation, and the age of the patient.

12 SCAPULAR (SHOULDER BLADE) FRACTURES

Scapular fractures are relatively uncommon injuries, accounting for approximately 1% of all fractures and 3-5% of fractures involving the shoulder girdle. Due to the scapula's strong bony structure and its protected position behind the rib cage, significant trauma is required to cause these fractures.

OUTLINE OF SCAPULAR FRACTURES:

Shoulder anatomy. Bones and joint capsule

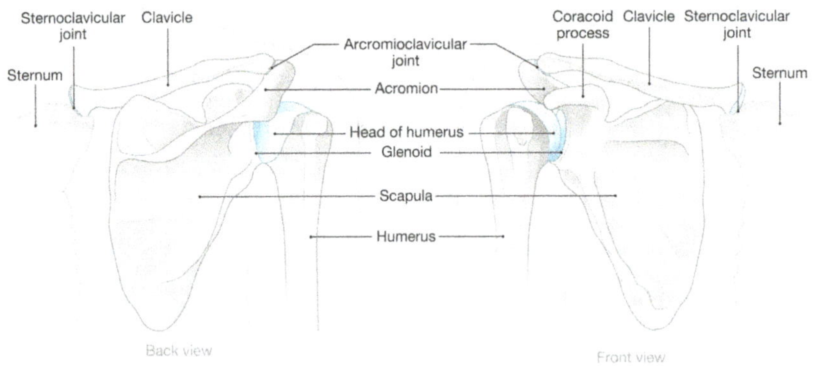

Fig. 12.1 Scapular Anatomy

ANATOMY INVOLVED

Body of the Scapula Is the most common site (50-60%) of Scapular fractures).

Scapular neck fractures comprises 25% of scapular fractures.

Acromion fractures represent 8-12% of cases of shoulder fractures..

The Glenoid portion of the **Scapula** involves the joint surface, and can be intra-articular (involving the glenoid fossa). This is very bad for the joint.

The coracoid process of the **Scapula** is less common but occurs in about 7-10% of scapular fractures.

Spine of the scapula fractures are rare, but can occur from direct trauma.

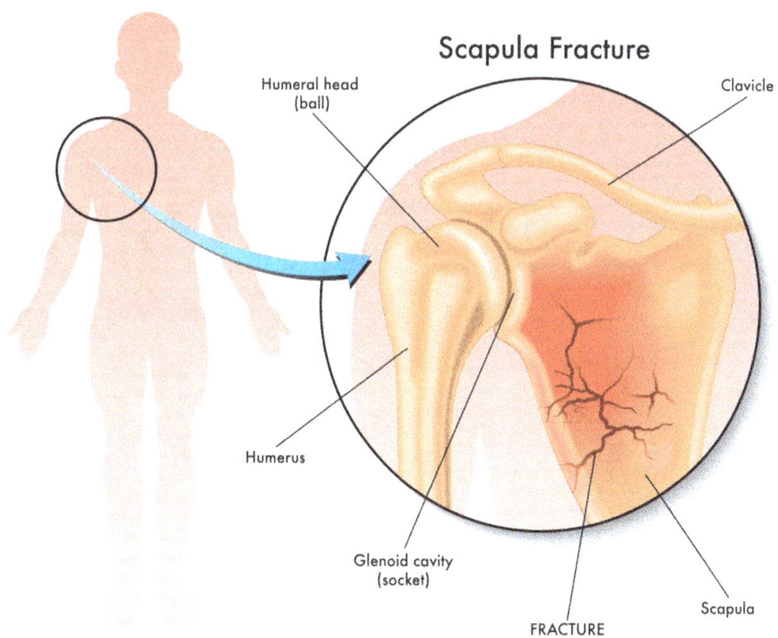

Fig. 12.2 Fracture of the Scapular Body

MECHANISM OF INJURY

High-energy trauma: The majority of scapular fractures are caused by high-energy mechanisms like motor vehicle accidents, falls from significant heights, or direct trauma (e.g., impact from contact sports).

Associated injuries: Because of the high force involved, scapular fractures often occur with other injuries like rib fractures, lung contusions, clavicle fractures, or injuries to the head, spine, and chest.

CLINICAL PRESENTATION

Pain and tenderness is localized pain around the scapula, especially with shoulder movement and is very common.

Swelling and bruising may be evident around the scapula.

Limited range of motion with shoulder movements is due to pain or structural disruption.

DIAGNOSIS

X-rays: Initial imaging is performed although the scapula can be difficult to visualize clearly.

CT scans: Often necessary for better evaluation, especially in complex or intra-articular fractures.

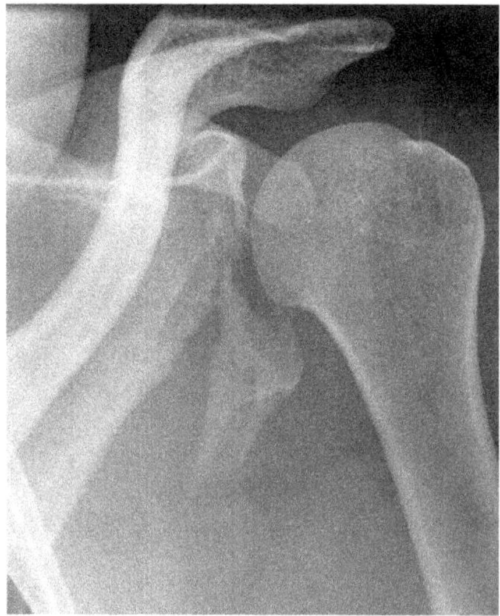

Fig. 12.3.1 X-ray of Scapular Neck Fracture

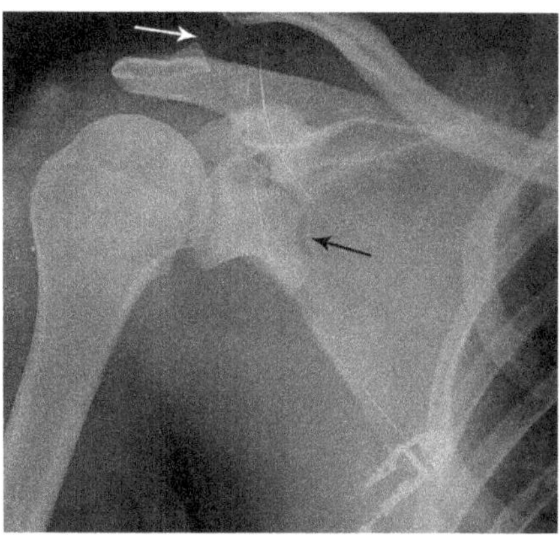

Fig. 12.3.2 X-ray Scapular Neck

DIAGNOSIS

Depending on which area of the Scapula the fracture is located dictates the treatment. As noted above there are fractures of the Body, Neck,Coracoid Process,Glenoid,Acromium, and spine.

MANAGEMENT

Non-operative treatment: The majority of scapular fractures (80-90%) can be treated non-surgically with immobilization (e.g., sling), rest, and rehabilitation.

Indicated for fractures with minimal displacement or extra-articular fractures.

Surgical treatment: Required for fractures involving the glenoid fossa (articular surface), significantly displaced fractures, or those associated with other injuries requiring surgical intervention (e.g., clavicle or rib fractures).

Open reduction internal fixation of the fractures is required for all of these injuries. Scapula is a deep bone with a great deal of neurovascular structure surrounding it and it is a very complex surgery only to be done some by someone that is experienced in these types of shoulder procedures. Each case is unique and the surgical approach has to be different internal fixation devices also have to be customized for this type of procedure

REHABILITATION

Early physical therapy focuses on restoring range of motion and strengthening surrounding muscles.

Return to full activity is typically seen within 6-12 weeks, depending on the severity and the treatment course.

Prognos is generally good with non-operative management for most fractures.

Surgical cases involving the Glenoid or displaced fractures may have a longer recovery and a risk of complications such as arthritis or shoulder instability.

CONCLUSION

Understanding the complexities of the shoulder, one of the most mobile and versatile joints in the human body, is crucial for anyone facing injury, surgery, or chronic pain. As we've explored throughout this guide, the shoulder's unique anatomy allows for an incredible range of motion but also makes it susceptible to various conditions and injuries.

Your journey to recovery or managing a shoulder condition is deeply personal. Whether you're an athlete eager to return to your sport, someone seeking relief from daily discomfort, or a patient preparing for surgery, knowledge is your greatest ally. By understanding the underlying causes of shoulder problems, the available treatment options, and the steps you can take to maintain shoulder health, you empower yourself to make informed decisions.

As you move forward, remember that healing takes time and effort. Stay proactive in your treatment, communicate openly with your healthcare providers, and don't hesitate to seek support when needed. Your commitment to your health and well-being is the key to achieving the best possible outcome.

Thank you for trusting this guide to assist you on your journey. Here's to a future filled with strength, mobility, and a pain-free life.

SUMMARY AND FINAL RECOMMENDATIONS

"Your Painful Shoulder" has taken you through a comprehensive exploration of the shoulder joint, its anatomy, common injuries, and the various treatment options available. Whether you're dealing with a rotator cuff tear, shoulder impingement, instability, arthritis, or other conditions, understanding the structure and function of the shoulder is the first step in your journey toward recovery.

KEY TAKEAWAYS:

Anatomy and Function:

The shoulder is an intricate joint that allows for a wide range of motion but is prone to instability and injury due to its complexity.

Key structures like the rotator cuff, labrum, and various tendons and ligaments play crucial roles in maintaining shoulder stability and function.

Common Shoulder Conditions:

Rotator Cuff Injuries: Often caused by overuse or trauma, these injuries can range from inflammation (tendinitis) to complete tears.

Shoulder Impingement: This occurs when shoulder tendons are compressed, leading to pain and limited mobility.

Shoulder Instability: This can result from dislocations or subluxations, where the joint moves out of its normal position.

Arthritis: Degenerative changes in the shoulder joint can lead to stiffness, pain, and reduced function over time.

Diagnostic and Treatment Options:

Accurate diagnosis through physical exams, imaging studies, and sometimes diagnostic injections is essential for effective treatment planning.

Non-Surgical Treatments: These include physical therapy, medications, injections, and activity modifications to relieve pain and restore function.

Surgical Options: For severe cases, surgical interventions like rotator cuff repair, labral repair, or shoulder replacement might be necessary. Understanding the risks, benefits, and recovery process is key to making an informed decision.

Rehabilitation and Recovery:

Rehabilitation is a critical component of recovery, whether you undergo surgery or pursue non-surgical treatments. A structured physical therapy program tailored to your specific condition can significantly enhance outcomes.

Patience and adherence to your rehab plan are vital, as shoulder recovery can be a gradual pro

Stay Informed: Knowledge is power. Continue educating yourself about your condition and treatment options. This will help you make confident decisions and advoc

Communicate with Your Healthcare Team: Open communication with your surgeon, physical therapist, and other healthcare providers is crucial. Don't hesitate to ask questions, express concerns, and seek clarification when needed.

Commit to Your Recovery: Whether through physical therapy, lifestyle modifications, or surgical recovery, your commitment will greatly influence your outcome. Follow your treatment plan diligently and maintain a positive mindset.

Prevent Future Issues: Incorporate shoulder-strengthening exercises, proper posture, and ergonomic adjustments into your daily routine to prevent re-injury or new problems.

ACKNOWLEDGMENTS

Without the expert help of Michael Silver, B.S., M.A., I would not have been able to produce this book. He is an expert in computer software, 3D imaging, and the manufacturing of medical models used by surgeons for training. With his training in anatomy, he was able to assist in editing this complex book and educated me on the best use of my time and knowledge. Thank you, Michael, for your time, expertise, and love. And, by the way, he is my son.

I would also like to acknowledge my wife, Lynnette, for her unwavering love and support throughout this writing process. Her devotion allowed me to focus on the task at hand for many months. I am also deeply grateful to my sister Sheryl, my daughter, Sophia, and granddaughter, Lily, for their love and encouragement. Likewise, my son, Stephen, his wife, Mary, and my other grandchildren, Ella and Felix, have provided me with endless support and love. My entire family has truly been a blessing in my life.

I would like to extend my gratitude to Sofía Castaño and Andres Herrera for their professional assistance in developing this book. Thanks also to the entire staff at Spine Publishing.

During my 46 years of orthopedic practice, and for over 20 of those years, I had two key personnel who were instrumental in patient care and organization. My office manager and nurse, Alicia Armas-Castrellon, LVN, was invaluable in keeping my practice running smoothly and ensuring patient satisfaction.

My other nurse, Jackie Moran, M.A., was exceptional in providing direct patient care and assisting me in numerous ways over the years. Their contributions were, in my opinion, invaluable to my ability to compile the experiences referenced in this book.

LIST OF FIGURES

3. SHOULDER DISLOCATION AND SUBLUXATION

4. SHOULDER IMPINGEMENT

5. LABRAL TEARS

6. FROZEN SHOULDER

7. COMMON CHALLENGES AND COMPLICATIONS IN ROTATOR CUFF SURGERY

8. ACROMIOCLAVICULAR (A-C) SEPARATIONS AND ARTHRITIS

9. CLAVICLE FRACTURES

10. ARTHRITIS OF THE SHOULDER JOINT

11. HUMERAL HEAD FRACTURES

12. SCAPULAR FRACTURES

Cases Courtesy of the Following	**Images**
Mr. Jeremy Granville-Chapman	2.9
Windsor Upper Limb .Com	5.2.1, 5.2.2, 5.2.3, 5.3, 5.4.1, 5.4.2, 5.4.3, 5.4.4, 8.4.1, 8.4.2, 11.3
Thomas Magee, Md Et Al Ajr 181 Nov 2003	7.3
Jack Porrino, Md Et Al Skel Radiol March 2020	8.2.1
Bernard Kempker, Md Et Al Crortho .Com	10.3
Cari Nierenberg Nejm Nov 15 2017	4.6
Joaquin Sanchez Sotelo, Md Shoulder.Elbow / .Org / 2016 / 09 / 19	11.9
Alessandro Castagna, Md Et Al Kssta Vol 25 / 7	8.2.3
Karas, Md Et Al Arthroscopy Techniques Issue 2 E319-324	6.4
Megan Severs Healthline A-C Joint Arthritis	8.3
Chul-Hyun Cho, Md Et Al Clinic N Orthopedics 2021 Vol 13 287-292	2.1
Sportsmedicine At Mayo Clinic *Sportsmedicine.Mayoclinic.Org*	7.4

www.ingramcontent.com/pod-product-compliance
Lightning Source LLC
Chambersburg PA
CBHW060922140726
47996CB00001B/349